Dear Reader,

One of the major objections I hear to starting a keto lifestyle is: "But I love carbs!" While I definitely understand that (who doesn't love a plate of nachos or a perfectly greasy pepperoni pizza?), unfortunately, most of those carbs don't love you back. The good news is that I'm here to offer you a solution: keto cycling.

The name sounds kind of fancy, but keto cycling is **actually simple**. Instead of restricting carbohydrates all the time, you alternate six days of low carbohydrates with one day of higher carbohydrates. It's the best of both worlds! One of my favorite things about keto cycling is that it feels less restrictive. And when a diet feels less restrictive, you're more likely to stick to it. Since the best diet is one that you can stick to, this middle ground works for many people.

In this book, I'll teach you all about keto cycling—what it is, the science behind why it works, the ways your body will benefit, and how to make your cycling schedule. I'll also explain the best types of carbohydrates to include on your high-carb days (spoiler alert: it's not nachos...sorry) and what makes these carbohydrates the best choices. After you get the lowdown on keto cycling, you'll move right into **300 recipes** that are organized into "keto" and "high-carb" chapters that you can use to design your keto cycling schedule and menu.

Whether you're new to keto cycling or a seasoned pro looking for some new recipes and inspiration, you'll find **something delicious to try**. And when you make the recipes, please reach out and tag me on *Instagram*. I'd love to see your creations! Thank you for picking up this book and making the commitment to change your health (and your life). I can't wait to hear from you!

In Health,
Lindsay Boyers, CHNC

Welcome to the Everything® Series!

These handy, accessible books give you all you need to tackle a difficult project, gain a new hobby, comprehend a fascinating topic, prepare for an exam, or even brush up on something you learned back in school but have since forgotten.

You can choose to read an Everything® book from cover to cover or just pick out the information you want from our four useful boxes: Questions, Facts, Alerts, and Essentials. We give you everything you need to know on the subject, but throw in a lot of fun stuff along the way too.

question	fact
Answers to common questions.	Important snippets of information.

alert	essential
Urgent warnings.	Quick handy tips.

We now have more than 600 Everything® books in print, spanning such wide-ranging categories as cooking, health, parenting, personal finance, wedding planning, word puzzles, and so much more. When you're done reading them all, you can finally say you know Everything®!

PUBLISHER Karen Cooper

MANAGING EDITOR Lisa Laing

COPY CHIEF Casey Ebert

ASSOCIATE PRODUCTION EDITOR Jo-Anne Duhamel

ACQUISITIONS EDITOR Zander Hatch

SENIOR DEVELOPMENT EDITOR Laura Daly

EVERYTHING® SERIES COVER DESIGNER Erin Alexander

THE

EVERYTHING®

KETO
CYCLING
COOKBOOK

LINDSAY BOYERS, CHNC

Author of *The Everything® Guide to the Ketogenic Diet*

**300 RECIPES FOR STARTING—AND
MAINTAINING—THE KETO LIFESTYLE**

ADAMS MEDIA

NEW YORK   LONDON   TORONTO   SYDNEY   NEW DELHI

To Joey.
Thank you for your unconditional support and for loving me as
I am while always gently encouraging me to be better.
You are the light at the end of my tunnel, and yet, you're so funny in the dark.
I love you so much.

Aadamsmedia

Adams Media
An Imprint of Simon & Schuster, Inc.
57 Littlefield Street
Avon, Massachusetts 02322

An Everything® Series Book.
Everything® and everything.com® are registered trademarks of Simon & Schuster, Inc.

First Adams Media trade paperback edition
October 2019

ADAMS MEDIA and colophon are trademarks of Simon & Schuster.

For information about special discounts for bulk purchases, please contact Simon & Schuster Special Sales at 1-866-506-1949 or business@simonandschuster.com.

The Simon & Schuster Speakers Bureau can bring authors to your live event. For more information or to book an event contact the Simon & Schuster Speakers Bureau at 1-866-248-3049 or visit our website at www.simonspeakers.com.

Interior design by Colleen Cunningham
Photographs by James Stefiuk
Chapter 1 image © Getty Images/samael334

Manufactured in the United States of America

10 9 8 7 6 5 4 3 2 1

Library of Congress Cataloging-in-Publication Data
Names: Boyers, Lindsay, author.
Title: The everything® keto cycling cookbook / Lindsay Boyers, CHNC, author of The everything® guide to the ketogenic diet.
Description: Avon, Massachusetts: Adams Media, 2019.
Series: Everything®.
Includes index.
Identifiers: LCCN 2019023021 | ISBN 9781507210598 (pb) | ISBN 9781507210604 (ebook)
Subjects: LCSH: Ketogenic diet. | Low-carbohydrate diet--Recipes. | Reducing diets--Recipes. | LCGFT: Cookbooks.
Classification: LCC RM237.73 .B692 2019 | DDC 641.5/6383--dc23
LC record available at https://lccn.loc.gov/2019023021

ISBN 978-1-5072-1059-8
ISBN 978-1-5072-1060-4 (ebook)

Contents

Introduction

The average American takes in more than 50 percent of their calories from carbohydrates. Most of these carbohydrates are in the form of high-glycemic carbohydrates, like sugar and wheat. While these types of carbs (like pizza, ice cream, and mac and cheese) may feel good while you're eating them, they have a lingering effect on your body. A diet that's too high in carbohydrates, especially the wrong types of carbohydrates, is a major risk factor for many chronic health issues. Researchers link diabetes, heart disease, infertility, macular degeneration, certain cancers, weight gain, and chronic inflammation (to name a few) back to eating too many carbohydrates.

One of the ways to avoid the potential negative impact of too many carbohydrates is to cut them almost completely out of your diet. Or, in other words, start following a standard keto diet, which restricts carbohydrates to around 5 to 10 percent of total calories. While this approach works really well for some people, others might need to consume a higher amount of carbs occasionally to feel their best. Enter the solution: keto cycling.

Keto cycling gives carbohydrate lovers the best of both worlds. You alternate between six days of really low carbohydrate intake and one day of a higher carbohydrate intake. This method of alternating between keto days and high-carb days keeps your body guessing about what types of foods to expect; and when your body doesn't know what's coming next, it turns into an efficient fat-burning machine. When you replenish your glycogen stores on your higher-carb days, you can increase the intensity of your workouts and favorably balance the hormones that increase metabolism and contribute to muscle growth. Then on your low-carb days, you'll deplete your glycogen stores and encourage your body to burn fat for energy.

Although you're given some leeway with the amount of carbs you're taking in, you still have to make educated choices on which types of carbohydrates are best. High-carb days aren't meant to be an excuse for stuffing yourself with simple carbohydrates, like donuts, pasta, and cookies. These types of carbohydrates can lead to poorly regulated insulin and blood sugar levels and chronic inflammation—the opposite of your health goals. Instead, you'll use your higher-carb days to eat low-glycemic carbohydrates that contribute to your overall health and micronutrient intake. The best types of carbohydrates are fruits and vegetables, like apples, berries, bananas, sweet potatoes, beets, butternut squash, and pumpkin, as well as brown rice, quinoa, and (soaked) beans.

From mouthwatering Cinnamon Waffles with Cinnamon Cream Cheese Icing to delectable Spinach and Feta–Stuffed Chicken Breasts, you'll find three hundred delicious dishes inside that the whole family will enjoy. Don't wait another day to start reducing the negative impacts of carbs on your body—let keto cycling help you regulate blood sugar, lower inflammation, lose weight, and feel great!

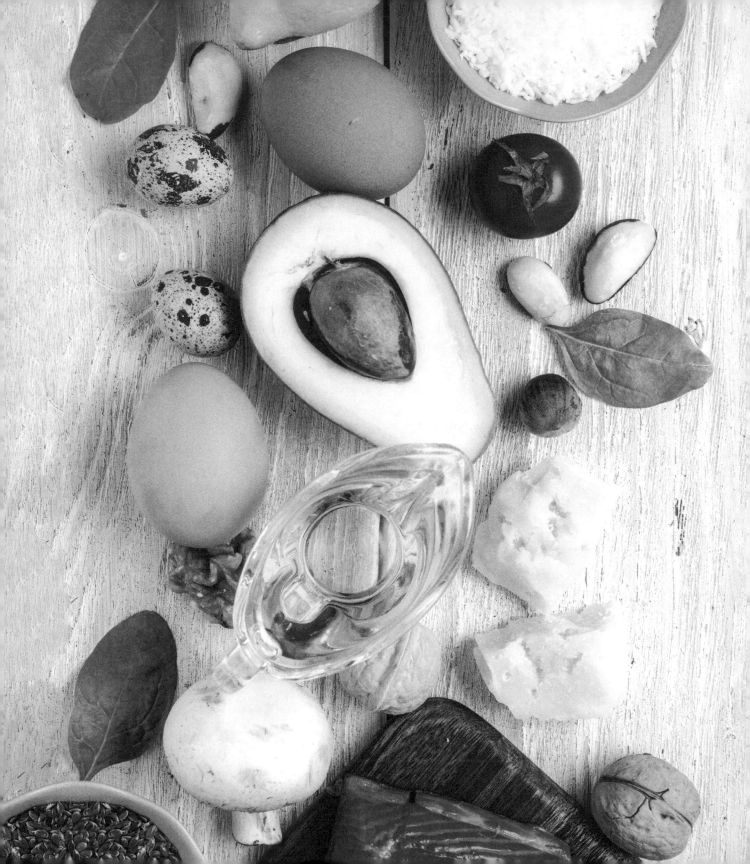

The Keto Cycling Lifestyle

The ketogenic diet is built around one major guideline: Restrict the amount of carbohydrates you eat and replace those carbohydrates with fat. Whether you're someone who's tried a standard ketogenic diet but couldn't stick to it (or didn't see the results you wanted), or you're just not ready or willing to give up carbohydrates entirely, or you're an athlete looking to boost your endurance and performance and increase muscle mass, you might find that adopting the keto cycling lifestyle is a good choice for you.

What Is Keto Cycling?

Keto cycling is a version of the ketogenic diet that combines several days of carbohydrate restriction with days of high carbohydrate intake. You'll cycle through two phases:

1. Five to six days of a standard keto diet (or a diet high in fat and low in carbs)
2. One to two days of a carb load phase (or a diet high in carbohydrates and low in fat)

With keto cycling, you get the ongoing health benefits of the low-carb foundation in the first phase (the standard keto diet) yet still get to enjoy nutritious carbs in the second phase (the carb load phase) from time to time.

> **alert**
>
> If you're pregnant or breastfeeding, you should avoid ketosis and fasting. If you have adrenal fatigue, thyroid dysfunction, diabetes, or any other hormone dysregulation, talk to your functional medicine doctor about whether keto cycling is right for you.

The Standard Keto Diet Phase

When you're keto cycling, you'll follow a standard keto diet most of the time to restrict carbohydrates enough that you kick your body into ketosis—a metabolic state in which your body burns fat for energy instead of carbohydrates.

The Science of Ketosis

Your body loves to use carbohydrates for energy. When you eat carbohydrates, they travel through your digestive system and are eventually broken down into a simple sugar called glucose, which makes its way into your bloodstream. The presence of glucose in your blood triggers a cascade of responses that starts with the release of insulin from the pancreas. Once insulin is released from the pancreas, it finds glucose and attaches to the simple sugar. Then, one of two things happen:

1. The insulin carries glucose to your cells, where your body uses it for immediate energy.
2. Your body converts the glucose to glycogen, which is then stored in your liver and muscles for the next time you need energy (like in between meals).

As long as you're regularly supplying your body with glucose (by eating carbohydrates), this cycle continues. When your body is relying on carbohydrates as its main energy source, it stores the fat you eat in your fat cells, and it stays there indefinitely.

The goal of the ketogenic diet, and the standard keto diet phase, is to restrict carbohydrate intake enough that it interrupts this metabolic process and your body has to use something else—fats—for energy.

Your body prefers using carbohydrates for energy, but in their absence, it will turn to fat for the fuel it needs. To turn fat into usable energy, the liver breaks it down into fatty acids and converts them into energy-rich substances called *ketones*. When you have ketones in your blood, you're in a state of ketosis—your body is burning fat for energy instead of carbohydrates.

> **fact**
>
> Your body has a limited ability to store carbohydrates. It uses the glucose it needs and then stores about twenty-four hours' worth of glycogen in the liver for use in between meals. On the other hand, your body's ability to store fat is endless. If your fat cells run out of room, your body will just make them bigger.

The Macronutrient Breakdown During the Standard Keto Diet Phase

The exact percentage of each macronutrient that you need during your standard keto diet phases varies from person to person. Play around with it to find out what works for you. Are you feeling good? Do you have energy? Are you reaching (or staying at) your ideal body weight? Can you get through your workouts effectively? The goal is to feel energized and healthy. If you feel sluggish and lightheaded and you're not able to lose any weight, you'll need to change up what you're doing.

In general, the range for each macronutrient on your standard keto diet phase is:

- 60–75 percent of calories from fat
- 15–30 percent of calories from protein
- 5–10 percent of calories from carbohydrates

The Carb Load Phase

After following a standard keto diet for five to six days, you'll jump into a carb load phase for the remaining days of the week. The goal of the carb load phase is to strategically supply your body with the carbohydrates it needs to refill your glycogen stores. This boosts energy, strength, and endurance and, ultimately, makes your body more efficient at burning fat.

The Science of the Carb Load Phase

Doesn't increasing carbohydrate intake in phase two of keto cycling kick you out of ketosis and defeat the entire purpose? Not if you do it strategically. When you eat carbohydrates, your glucose levels go up and, as a result, your insulin levels also increase. Insulin attaches to the glucose and carries it to your liver, but it also travels to your muscles, which have insulin receptors.

When the insulin reaches your muscles, it allows glucose and amino acids like creatine, which supplies your body with energy, to enter the muscle cells. From there, insulin starts a biochemical reaction that simultaneously increases the building of new muscle while decreasing muscle and protein breakdown.

An increase in insulin also triggers the blood vessels to dilate, or open up, which allows more blood to get to the muscles. This blood carries important muscle-building nutrients like oxygen, amino acids, and glucose with it.

When insulin increases and carries glucose to the muscles, it also replenishes depleted muscle glycogen stores. This muscle glycogen significantly improves your energy, strength, and endurance, which makes it especially useful during exercise.

So how do you avoid the fat-storing potential of insulin while also taking advantage of its ability to boost energy and muscle? By alternating days of carbohydrate restriction with days of high carbohydrate intake, or keto cycling.

The Macronutrient Breakdown During the Carb Load Phase

The breakdown of the carb load phase is almost the exact opposite of the standard keto diet phase. Instead of getting the majority of your calories from fat, you'll be limiting your fat intake and taking in mostly carbohydrates.

Typically, a carb load phase looks like this:

- 5–10 percent of calories from fat
- 15–20 percent of calories from protein
- 70 percent of calories from carbohydrates

Benefits of a Keto Cycling Diet

A basic ketogenic diet can:

- Speed up weight loss
- Increase energy
- Improve body composition
- Decrease inflammation
- Improve brain function
- Lower blood sugar levels and improve insulin sensitivity

Research into whether the keto diet can influence certain diseases is ongoing and incomplete, but early studies show that it may:

- Improve risk factors for heart disease
- Slow tumor growth for some cancers
- Reduce symptoms of Alzheimer's and slow disease progression
- Reduce frequency and severity of seizures in those with epilepsy

Keto cycling offers all these benefits, plus it adds *more* benefits that aren't seen with a ketogenic diet alone. Let's look at those benefits.

- **Promotes metabolic flexibility.** Metabolic flexibility describes your body's ability to respond and adapt to changes, such as switching between burning fat and burning carbs for energy. In simple terms, when you have metabolic flexibility, your body is really efficient. When you're metabolically inflexible, you feel fatigued, you experience a midday crash, you need snacks to sustain your energy, and you rely on stimulants, like coffee, to get through the day. Keto cycling can help improve metabolic flexibility by teaching your body how to use fats for fuel and by using carbohydrates strategically to increase glycogen stores.

- **Increases production of natural anabolic hormones.** Keto cycling can increase testosterone, growth hormone, and insulin-like growth factor 1, or IGF-1—three anabolic hormones that help increase muscle growth, improve strength, and enhance collagen production. Research shows that eating a lot of fat can increase testosterone and growth hormone, but it tends to lower IGF-1. On the other hand, IGF-1 increases after a period of increased carbohydrate intake. Combining high-fat, low-carbohydrate days with lower-fat, high-carbohydrate days can target all the anabolic hormones.
- **Improves exercise performance.** Although you can use fat for energy during moderate exercise, high-intensity exercise puts increased demands on the body. If you don't have any stored muscle glycogen, it can negatively affect your performance during high-intensity and endurance exercises. Keto cycling provides just enough carbohydrates to refill your muscle glycogen stores so that you can use them for energy, but not so much that excess glucose is stored as fat.
- **Offers high potential for long-term adherence.** Even with all the known benefits of the keto diet, sticking to it

can be difficult. Because carbohydrates are your body's preferred energy source, your body doesn't like to be without them, especially at first. For some, these cravings go away pretty quickly. For others, they're persistent and make sticking with a keto diet for the long term nearly impossible.

fact

Fiber-rich foods, which also tend to be higher in carbohydrates, promote the growth of good bacteria in your gut. When your gut bacteria are balanced, your mood improves as well as your health. Sometimes called the "second brain," the gut is a collection of more than one hundred million neurons. Formally called the *enteric nervous system*, it has its own reflexes and senses. In fact, 90 percent of the information in the primary nerve in your gut (the *vagus nerve*) is carried from the gut to the brain, and not the other way around.

If you fall into the latter category, keto cycling provides a little more flexibility. Because you can eat some high-carb foods that you're missing during your carb load phase, the diet may be more sustainable, so you can stick with it.

There's also research that shows that keto cycling can improve sleep, boost immune function, and promote a healthier balance of bacteria in your gut. You tend to take in more fiber on a keto cycling diet than you do on a standard keto diet. This helps reduce constipation.

Choosing High-Quality Carbs

When it comes to carbs, it's all about quality. It's not enough to simply focus on the amount of carbohydrates you're taking in; you need to make sure that you're eating high-quality complex carbohydrates that contribute to your overall nutrient intake.

What Are Complex Carbohydrates?

Although all types of carbohydrates are turned into glucose eventually, complex carbohydrates move through your body slowly and take longer to digest than their counterpart: simple carbohydrates. Simple carbohydrates contain sugars in their most basic forms. Because the body doesn't have to break down these sugars to absorb them, the sugars move into the bloodstream right away. Complex carbohydrates, on the other hand, are held together by long, complex chains of sugar molecules that the body has to break apart into their simplest forms before it can absorb them.

> **essential**
>
> As a general rule, complex carbohydrates are also higher in nutrients, like fiber, vitamins, minerals, phytonutrients, and antioxidants, than simple carbohydrates. When you include a variety of complex carbohydrates in your diet, you'll also increase the variety of nutrients you're taking in. Of course, these nutrients work together to keep you healthy, but they're also vital to keeping your metabolism running efficiently.

Because your digestive system has to break down complex carbohydrates into simpler sugars before they can enter your bloodstream, your blood sugar and insulin levels stay fairly low and consistent, even when taking in more carbs on your higher-carb days. But when you eat simple carbohydrates, your digestive system doesn't have to spend any time breaking them down, so they quickly move right into your bloodstream, causing spikes (and then resulting crashes) in blood sugar and insulin. These spikes and crashes can trigger your body to store extra fat.

Healthy Carb Choices

The goal with keto cycling is to provide your body with carbohydrates in a way that replenishes your glycogen stores but prevents surges in blood sugar and insulin levels. On your high-carb days, choose:

- Sweet potatoes
- Butternut squash
- Beets
- Berries
- Bananas
- Apples
- Pineapple
- Mango
- Brown rice
- Wild rice
- Quinoa
- Lentils
- Beans

Avoid these types of carbohydrates:

- Refined grains (white bread, white rice, white pasta, pizza)
- Sweets (cookies, cakes, candy)
- Sugar-sweetened beverages (soda, fruit juice, sports drinks, iced teas, lemonade)

Tips for Getting Back Into Ketosis

The amount of time it takes to get back into ketosis after your carb load phase varies, but there are things you can do to speed up your return to a fat-burning state.

- On your last day of your high-carb phase, stop eating at 6 p.m. When you enter a fasting state, your body breaks down stored glycogen more quickly so you can switch to burning fat for fuel.
- On Day One of your standard keto diet phase, perform a high-intensity exercise for 30 to 60 minutes on an empty stomach immediately after waking up.
- On Day Two of your standard keto diet phase, perform a moderate-intensity exercise for 30 to 60 minutes on an empty stomach immediately after waking up.

These tips can help your body transition back into a fat-burning state as soon as possible.

Designing a Keto Cycling Schedule

If you've been following a standard ketogenic diet and are ready to transition to keto cycling, you may be able to dive right in. If you're new to keto, ease in slowly. Start by cutting out simple carbohydrates and sources of refined sugar, like soda, desserts, bread, and sugar in your coffee. After a week, reduce your intake of fruit, whole grains, beans, and legumes for another week. Once you're used to restricting the obvious sources of carbohydrates, transition to a standard ketogenic diet, which also restricts high-carbohydrate vegetables, like sweet potatoes and beets.

Start with Standard Keto

Before starting keto cycling, it's best to follow a standard ketogenic diet for a period of four to six weeks before introducing high-carb days. This keto period helps your body convert over to fat burning so that when you reintroduce carbohydrates, you'll be more likely to use them efficiently.

Determining the High-Carb Days

You'll have to decide how many high-carb days you want to include and which days will be your high-carb days. If you are a bodybuilder or an endurance athlete or if muscle building is your goal, then you may want to shoot for two high-carb days. If you exercise regularly, but moderately, or your goal is weight loss, it's likely you'd do better with one high-carb day.

Plan the Timing of Your Cycles

After you've decided on your number, you need to figure out your timing. Most people choose to do their standard keto diet phase during the week and their carb load phase on the weekend; but what works best for you depends on your schedule and personal preference.

Cycling Tips

Don't just focus on the quantity of fats and carbohydrates. Other factors are also vital to your success:

- **Choose your carbs wisely:** High-carb days aren't an excuse for bingeing on the pizza, cookies, and syrup-covered pancakes that you've been missing. Focus on low-glycemic, nutrient-dense carbs like starchy vegetables, fruits, certain whole grains, and fiber-rich beans.
- **Stay hydrated:** Drink plenty of water and make sure you're getting enough electrolytes. You can make your own electrolyte drinks with Himalayan salt and magnesium and calcium powders, or you can purchase high-quality electrolyte supplements. Stay away from sports drinks, even the sugar-free versions.
- **Manage your stress:** Keto and intermittent fasting are both stressors. Although they're intentional, good stressors, sometimes your body can't tell the difference. Managing your stress is a vital component of the keto cycling lifestyle. Try meditation, yoga, reading, writing, and indulging the creative part of your brain until you find a stress management program that works for you.
- **Get adequate sleep:** A lack of sleep disrupts your hunger hormones. When you're tired, your body has a hard time deciding when it's full and when it's hungry. It also has a hard time managing stress hormones. Get on a healthy sleep schedule, like 10 p.m. to 6 a.m. Keep electronics and pets out of the room, turn off lights, and make the room really dark.
- **Make sure you're pooping:** It's become taboo to talk about poop even though everyone does it. Constipation is one of the most common digestive complaints. It isn't just uncomfortable; it's a major problem. Your digestive system is one of your primary routes of detoxification. If it's clogged up, your body isn't able to effectively remove toxins. Make sure your digestive system is moving properly. You can try increasing fiber, drinking more water, taking magnesium supplements, exercising, going to the bathroom as soon as you feel the urge, and reducing your stress.

When you're first starting out, it can take a little while until you find a cycling schedule that works for you and an exercise plan that fits into your lifestyle. You may have to adjust your macros—more than once—and play around with different types of carbohydrates to find out which ones make you feel the best. Don't get discouraged with this trial and error—instead, have fun with it. Putting in this work in the beginning will make everything easier as you go.

Look through the recipes in this book to get yourself excited at all your options. Relish in all the delicious foods you can enjoy every day instead of focusing on what you "can't" have. Plan favorite dishes on your carb-loading days so you can look forward to them. Find friends and family members who will encourage you on your journey, and share your successes with them. You'll be feeling—and looking—great in no time!

CHAPTER 2

Keto Breakfast

Avocado Everything "Bagels"

These cream cheese–stuffed avocados give you the distinct flavors of an everything bagel but without all the carbs. You won't even miss the bread!

1 large avocado

2 tablespoons cream cheese, softened

2 teaspoons dried chives

1 tablespoon everything bagel seasoning

1   Cut avocado in half lengthwise and remove the pit.

2   Combine cream cheese and chives in a small bowl and mix until incorporated.

3   Scoop 1 tablespoon of cream cheese mixture into the center of each avocado half. Sprinkle ½ tablespoon seasoning on top of each avocado. Serve immediately.

Iced Matcha Lattes

If you prefer your lattes hot, combine all ingredients in a saucepan over low heat and whisk until blended. The full-fat coconut milk will help you meet your macronutrient goals during the keto phase.

1 teaspoon matcha powder

1 tablespoon granulated erythritol

1 teaspoon vanilla extract

2 teaspoons vanilla MCT oil powder

2 cups full-fat coconut milk

1 tablespoon grass-fed collagen powder

1   Add all ingredients, except collagen, to a blender and blend until smooth. Add collagen and pulse until just incorporated.

2   Pour over ice and serve immediately.

Keto English Muffins

These Keto English Muffins are delicious toasted and topped with butter or any nut or seed butter. They also make a great base for egg sandwiches. You can whip up a few of them at a time and store them in an airtight container in the refrigerator for 1 week or freeze them for up to 2 months and eat them when you're ready.

2 tablespoons no-sugar-added creamy almond butter

1 tablespoon grass-fed butter

2 tablespoons paleo flour

½ teaspoon baking powder

1 tablespoon full-fat coconut milk

1 large egg, lightly beaten

SERVES 2	
Per Serving:	
Calories	224
Fat	19g
Protein	7g
Sodium	37mg
Fiber	2g
Carbohydrates	7g
Net Carbs	5g
Sugar	1g

1 Preheat oven to 350°F. Spray four wells of a muffin top pan with coconut oil spray.

2 Combine almond butter and butter in a small microwave-safe bowl and microwave for 30 seconds. Stir until smooth.

3 Combine paleo flour and baking powder in a small bowl and stir until incorporated. Add milk and egg and stir until combined.

4 Pour flour mixture into almond butter mixture and stir until smooth.

5 Pour equal amounts of mixture in each prepared well. Bake for 12 minutes or until set. Remove from oven and allow to cool. Toast to desired doneness before serving.

Cinnamon Waffles with Cinnamon Cream Cheese Icing

SERVES 2

Per Serving:

Calories	304
Fat	26g
Protein	12g
Sodium	318mg
Fiber	3g
Carbohydrates	18g
Net Carbs	3g
Sugar	2g

WHAT IS MCT OIL POWDER?

Medium-chain triglycerides, or MCTs, are fatty acids that help stabilize blood sugar, increase production of ketones, reduce inflammation, boost metabolism, and improve brain function. They're found in high amounts in coconut products and palm oil. MCT oil powder is a supplemental form of MCT oil that gives you all the benefits of MCTs in a powdered form that's easy to incorporate into meals, fat bombs, and smoothies when you need to increase the fat content.

In addition to the cream cheese icing, you can top these waffles with monk fruit–sweetened maple-flavored syrup or some melted no-sugar-added almond butter.

6 tablespoons blanched almond flour

2 tablespoons granulated erythritol, divided

¼ teaspoon baking soda

1 teaspoon vanilla MCT oil powder

1 teaspoon ground cinnamon, divided

2 large eggs

1 teaspoon vanilla extract, divided

2 ounces cream cheese, softened

1 Preheat waffle iron.

2 Combine almond flour, 1 tablespoon erythritol, baking soda, MCT oil powder, and ¾ teaspoon cinnamon in a medium bowl.

3 Whisk together eggs and ¾ teaspoon vanilla extract in a small bowl. Fold eggs into dry ingredients.

4 Pour batter into waffle iron and allow to cook according to waffle iron manufacturer directions.

5 While waffle is cooking, combine cream cheese, remaining erythritol, remaining cinnamon, and remaining vanilla extract in a separate small bowl and beat until smooth.

6 Remove waffle from waffle iron and cut in half. Spread icing on top. Serve immediately.

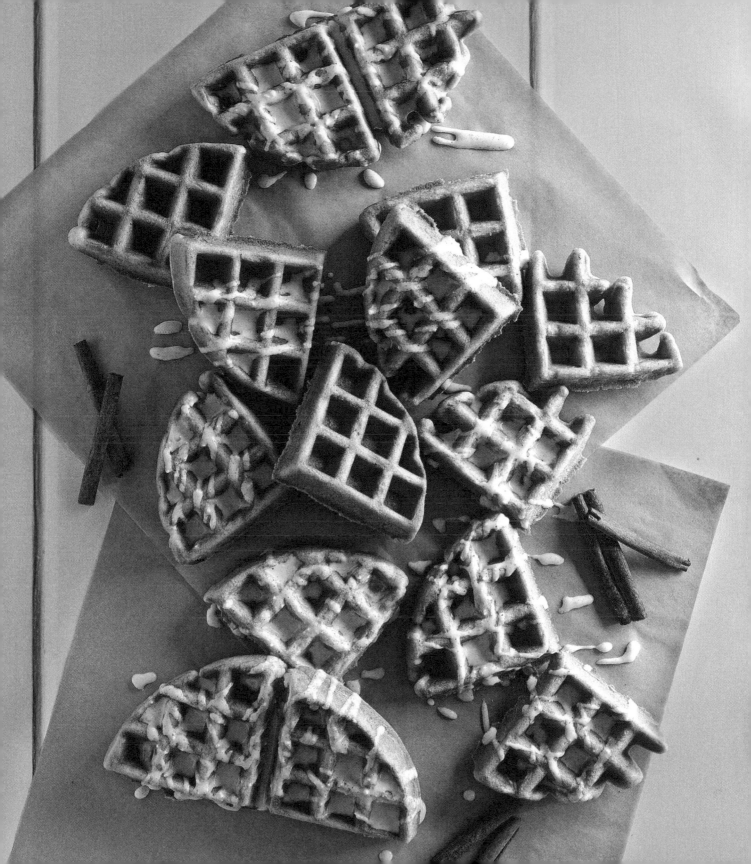

Egg, Spinach, and Feta–Stuffed Peppers

Stuffed peppers aren't just for dinner. These Egg, Spinach, and Feta–Stuffed Peppers help fill you up while adding a boost of vitamins and minerals to your breakfast so you can start your day off on the right foot.

1 large red bell pepper, halved lengthwise and seeded

4 large eggs, lightly beaten

¼ cup full-fat coconut milk

4 slices prosciutto, chopped

¼ cup chopped spinach

½ cup crumbled feta cheese

1 tablespoon dried chives

½ teaspoon sea salt

¼ teaspoon ground black pepper

1 Preheat oven to 400°F.

2 Place bell peppers cut side up in an 8" × 8" baking dish and bake for 5 minutes.

3 While peppers are cooking, whisk together eggs and coconut milk. Stir in remaining ingredients.

4 Pour equal amounts of egg mixture into each pepper half. Bake for 30 minutes or until eggs are set.

5 Remove from oven and allow to cool slightly. Serve warm.

Vanilla Cinnamon Pancakes

Full-fat coconut milk, which typically comes in a can, contains a higher fat percentage than the coconut milk beverages you find in a carton. Try to use this kind of coconut milk whenever possible. It's not only more keto-friendly; it also has minimal ingredients without a lot of additives.

¾ cup blanched almond flour

¼ teaspoon baking soda

¾ teaspoon ground cinnamon

⅛ teaspoon sea salt

1 teaspoon vanilla MCT oil powder

2 tablespoons granulated erythritol

2 large eggs

¼ cup full-fat coconut milk

2 teaspoons grass-fed butter, melted

1 teaspoon vanilla extract

⅛ teaspoon apple cider vinegar

2 tablespoons grass-fed butter

SERVES 2	
Per Serving:	
Calories	505
Fat	47g
Protein	15g
Sodium	367mg
Fiber	5g
Carbohydrates	21g
Net Carbs	4g
Sugar	2g

1 Combine almond flour, baking soda, cinnamon, salt, MCT oil powder, and erythritol in a small bowl.

2 In a medium bowl, whisk together eggs, coconut milk, melted butter, vanilla, and apple cider vinegar.

3 Fold dry ingredients into wet ingredients and stir until just combined.

4 Heat butter in a medium skillet over medium-low heat. Drop a ¼ cup of batter into the center of the skillet and cook for 3 minutes or until batter starts to bubble, then flip and cook for another 2 minutes. Repeat until batter is gone.

5 Serve immediately.

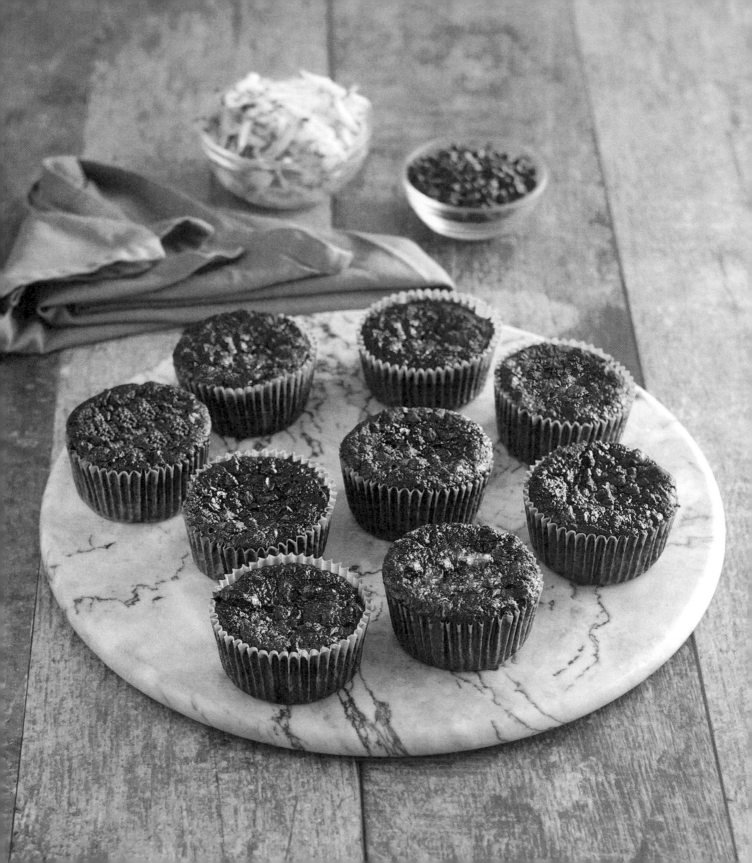

Chocolate Zucchini Muffins

These delicious muffins can help curb carb cravings in your keto phase, and they have added nutritional benefits too. The water content and fiber in the zucchini will help keep your digestion regular and blood sugar levels steady, and you'll also get some sweetness from the chocolate chips. They will freeze for up to 2 months, too, so you can make a couple batches in advance and save them for later.

½ cup coconut flour

⅓ cup unsweetened cocoa powder

1 teaspoon instant coffee granules

½ cup golden monk fruit sweetener

1 teaspoon baking soda

1 teaspoon baking powder

¼ teaspoon sea salt

¼ cup grass-fed butter, melted

4 large eggs

1 teaspoon vanilla extract

2 cups shredded zucchini, strained

½ cup stevia-sweetened chocolate chips

1 Preheat oven to 350°F. Line each well of a muffin tin with paper liners.

2 Combine coconut flour, cocoa, coffee granules, sweetener, baking soda, baking powder, and salt in a large mixing bowl.

3 Combine remaining ingredients, except chocolate chips, in a medium bowl.

4 Fold wet ingredients into dry ingredients, stirring just enough to incorporate ingredients. Stir in chocolate chips.

5 Pour equal amounts of batter into each well. Bake for 12 minutes or until a toothpick inserted in the center comes out clean.

6 Remove from oven and allow to cool for 5 minutes. Remove muffins from tin and transfer to a cooling rack. Cool completely before storing in an airtight container at room temperature for up to 1 week.

SERVES 12 (MAKES 12 MUFFINS)

Per Serving:

Calories	136
Fat	9g
Protein	4g
Sodium	183mg
Fiber	3g
Carbohydrates	19g
Net Carbs	8g
Sugar	1g

WHAT IS MONK FRUIT?

Monk fruit is a melon native to China and Thailand. Monk fruit extracts are natural, low-glycemic sweeteners that have zero calories or carbohydrates, so they don't raise your blood sugar. Monk fruit extract is typically combined with other sweeteners and erythritol; this blend can be swapped 1:1 with sugar. For recipes that call for monk fruit sweetener, make sure you're using a *blend* instead of pure extract, which is up to 250 times sweeter.

Egg and Sausage Pepper Rings

SERVES 2

Per Serving:

Calories	413
Fat	35g
Protein	19g
Sodium	1,332mg
Fiber	2g
Carbohydrates	6g
Net Carbs	4g
Sugar	4g

BREAKFAST SAUSAGE SEASONING

This breakfast sausage seasoning gives you all the flavor of sage breakfast sausage without any added sugars or artificial ingredients. You can make a big batch of this seasoning mix and keep it in an airtight container in your cabinet until you're ready to use it (it will keep for 6 months). Mix 1½ teaspoons dried sage, 1 teaspoon salt, 1 teaspoon ground black pepper, ¼ teaspoon dried marjoram, and ⅛ teaspoon crushed red pepper with 1 pound of ground pork.

When choosing your breakfast sausage, check your labels carefully! A lot of breakfast sausages have added sugar. If you can't find one that's suitable for your keto diet, ask your butcher to make you a sugar-free version or make your own with ground pork and a seasoning mix.

1 large red bell pepper
4 large eggs
½ teaspoon sea salt
¼ teaspoon ground black pepper
1 teaspoon dried chives

¼ pound no-sugar-added breakfast sausage
2 tablespoons butter-flavored coconut oil
2 tablespoons shredded Parmesan cheese

1 Cut top and bottom off bell pepper and remove seeds and membranes. Cut pepper in half widthwise. Finely dice pepper left from the top and bottom pieces and put in a medium mixing bowl.

2 Add eggs, salt, black pepper, and chives to diced peppers and whisk to combine. Set aside.

3 Heat medium skillet over medium heat and add breakfast sausage to pan. Cook until no longer pink, about 7 minutes.

4 Remove sausage from pan and set aside. Add coconut oil to pan.

5 Once coconut oil is hot, place peppers in pan and cook for 2 minutes, flip, and cook another 2 minutes.

6 Pour equal amounts of egg mixture into each pepper ring and sprinkle sausage on top. Cook until egg is almost set, about 4 minutes.

7 Sprinkle Parmesan cheese on top of pepper rings and cook until cheese starts to melt, another 2 minutes. Use a spatula to remove pepper rings from pan and serve immediately.

Chocolate Coffee Chia Pudding

If you prefer thinner pudding, stir in more coconut milk.

½ cup chilled brewed coffee

⅓ cup full-fat coconut milk

1 tablespoon no-sugar-added sunflower seed butter

1 teaspoon vanilla extract

3 tablespoons stevia-sweetened maple-flavored syrup

1 tablespoon unsweetened cocoa powder

⅛ teaspoon sea salt

¼ cup chia seeds

SERVES 2	
Per Serving:	
Calories	291
Fat	23g
Protein	9g
Sodium	258mg
Fiber	14g
Carbohydrates	20g
Net Carbs	6g
Sugar	1g

1 Combine all ingredients except chia seeds in a blender. Blend until smooth.

2 Pour equal amounts of mixture into two 16-ounce Mason jars. Add half the chia seeds to each jar and cover. Shake to combine.

3 Refrigerate for 4 hours or until pudding is set. Serve cold.

Coconut Cereal

This cereal is like oatmeal, but without all the carbohydrates.

1 tablespoon grass-fed butter

½ cup unsweetened coconut flakes

1 cup unsweetened vanilla almond milk

⅓ cup full-fat coconut milk

1 cup water

2 tablespoons coconut flour

1 tablespoon flaxseed meal

1 tablespoon chia seeds

1 tablespoon vanilla MCT oil powder

2 tablespoons granulated erythritol

2 tablespoons crushed walnuts

SERVES 2	
Per Serving:	
Calories	436
Fat	42g
Protein	7g
Sodium	135mg
Fiber	10g
Carbohydrates	28g
Net Carbs	6g
Sugar	2g

1 Heat butter in a medium saucepan over medium heat. Add coconut flakes and cook for 3 minutes, stirring constantly. Add almond milk, coconut milk, and water and stir to combine.

2 Increase heat to high and bring to a boil. Remove from heat and stir in remaining ingredients. Divide into two bowls and serve immediately.

Buffalo Chicken Egg Cups

SERVES 12	
Per Serving:	
Calories	101
Fat	6g
Protein	11g
Sodium	510mg
Fiber	0g
Carbohydrates	1g
Net Carbs	1g
Sugar	0g

Buffalo chicken and egg may not be a pair that you're used to seeing, but they should be! The two come together really nicely to form a high-protein keto breakfast on the go.

12 large eggs

1 teaspoon sea salt

¼ teaspoon ground black pepper

2 tablespoons dried chives

1 (9.75-ounce) can cooked chicken breast

⅓ cup Frank's RedHot Original Cayenne Pepper Sauce

¼ cup shredded Cheddar cheese

1 Preheat oven to 350°F. Spray each well of a muffin tin with coconut oil spray.

2 Whisk eggs, salt, pepper, and chives together in a large mixing bowl. Combine chicken and hot sauce in a medium bowl and toss to coat.

3 Pour equal amounts of egg mixture into each well of the muffin tin. Spoon chicken mixture evenly on top. Sprinkle cheese on top.

4 Bake for 15 minutes or until eggs are set. Remove from oven and allow to cool slightly. Serve warm.

5 Keep leftover egg cups refrigerated, and eat within 2 days.

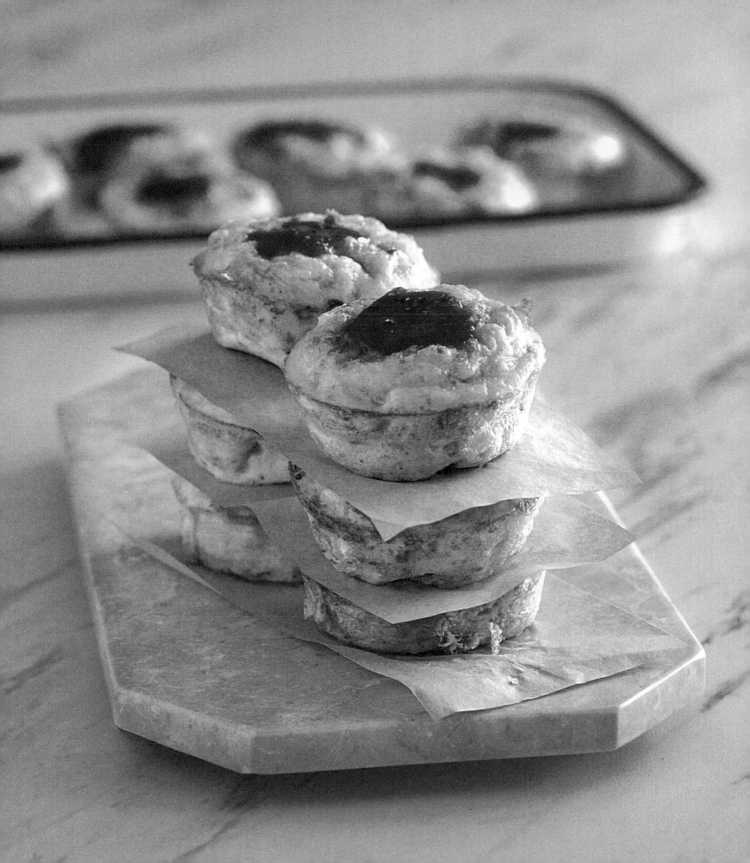

Chocolate Chip Banana Muffins

A PALEO FLOUR BREAKDOWN

Paleo flour typically contains a mixture of almond flour, coconut flour, and a thickener, like tapioca starch and arrowroot starch. You can substitute it in a 1:1 ratio in most recipes that call for all-purpose flour. Delicate recipes, like cakes, may require a different substitution. Make sure to read nutrition labels and carbohydrate counts when choosing which paleo flour you use, though. Some of them contain potato starch, which can increase the carbohydrate count.

These Chocolate Chip Banana Muffins call for banana extract to keep the carbohydrate count low, but if you're making them on one of your higher-carb days, you can add half of a small ripe banana for extra banana flavor and some added sweetness.

½ cup unsweetened almond milk

3 large eggs

⅓ cup grass-fed butter, melted

2 teaspoons banana extract

¼ cup granulated erythritol

2 cups paleo flour

1 teaspoon baking powder

½ cup stevia-sweetened chocolate chips

1 Preheat oven to 350°F. Line each well of a muffin tin with paper liners.

2 Whisk together almond milk, eggs, butter, and banana extract in a medium bowl.

3 In a separate medium bowl, combine erythritol, flour, and baking powder. Fold dry ingredients into wet ingredients and stir until just combined. Stir in chocolate chips.

4 Pour equal amounts of batter into each well and bake for 15 minutes or until a toothpick inserted in the center comes out clean.

5 Remove from oven and allow to cool for 5 minutes. Remove muffins from muffin tin and transfer to a cooling rack. Allow to cool completely before storing.

Waffled Omelet

Did you know you can use a waffle maker to make omelets? Well, you can; and it's a snap to make them this way, so give it a try.

2 large eggs

2 tablespoons full-fat coconut milk

1 tablespoon shredded white Cheddar cheese

1 tablespoon chopped spinach

1 tablespoon chopped broccoli

1 tablespoon chopped mushrooms

¼ teaspoon onion salt

⅛ teaspoon ground black pepper

SERVES 1	
Per Serving:	
Calories	231
Fat	18g
Protein	15g
Sodium	646mg
Fiber	0g
Carbohydrates	2g
Net Carbs	2g
Sugar	1g

1 Preheat waffle iron.

2 Combine all ingredients in a medium bowl and whisk until incorporated.

3 Pour egg mixture into waffle iron and cook for 5 minutes or until eggs are set. Remove from waffle iron and serve immediately.

Almond Cream Cheese Pancakes

These pancakes give you a healthy dose of fat with all the warm fuzziness of the traditional comfort food.

½ cup blanched almond flour

4 ounces cream cheese, softened

3 large eggs, lightly beaten

1½ teaspoons granulated erythritol

⅛ teaspoon sea salt

½ teaspoon baking powder

2 tablespoons grass-fed butter

SERVES 2	
Per Serving:	
Calories	548
Fat	50g
Protein	18g
Sodium	537mg
Fiber	3g
Carbohydrates	11g
Net Carbs	5g
Sugar	4g

1 Combine all ingredients except butter in a food processor and process until smooth.

2 Heat butter in a large skillet over medium heat. Drop batter by ¼-cupfuls onto hot skillet. When batter starts to bubble, flip over and cook for an additional 2 minutes.

3 Repeat until all the batter is gone. Serve warm.

Zucchini Fritters

SERVES 4	
Per Serving:	
Calories	141
Fat	9g
Protein	4g
Sodium	291mg
Fiber	4g
Carbohydrates	12g
Net Carbs	8g
Sugar	4g

SWEATING THE ZUCCHINI

Allowing zucchini to sit in salt for 30 minutes (which you'll do in the first step) helps draw out excess water so that you can squeeze it out before cooking certain recipes. This helps reduce moisture and ensures that you won't have a soggy finished product. You can do this with other watery vegetables, like sweet potatoes and spaghetti squash too.

When planning out your breakfast menu for the week, keep in mind that these fritters require you to "sweat" the zucchini for 30 minutes before cooking. It's an important step, so make the extra time in your routine or save these for a morning when you have more time to cook.

2 large zucchini
½ teaspoon sea salt
2½ tablespoons coconut flour
2 tablespoons arrowroot powder
1 large egg, lightly beaten
½ teaspoon onion powder
½ teaspoon garlic powder
½ teaspoon ground black pepper
2 tablespoons butter-flavored coconut oil

1 Shred zucchini using a cheese grater or the shredding attachment of a food processor. Transfer zucchini to a strainer and sprinkle with salt. Toss to coat. Let zucchini sit for 30 minutes to let excess water drain out.

2 After 30 minutes, use a cheesecloth or a nut milk bag to squeeze out as much excess moisture as you can.

3 Combine remaining ingredients, except coconut oil, in a large bowl and stir to combine. Add zucchini and stir well.

4 Heat coconut oil in a large skillet over medium heat. Scoop zucchini mixture by the tablespoonful into hot skillet. Press down to flatten into rounds. Repeat until skillet is full. Cook for 3 minutes or until zucchini starts to brown. Flip and cook on the other side for another 3 minutes.

5 Place zucchini on paper towel–lined plate to absorb excess oil.

6 Repeat until all fritters are cooked. Serve immediately.

Zucchini Egg Cups

These muffin tin treats are a great grab-and-go breakfast. When choosing ham, check your ingredient lists. Many have added sweeteners that up the carbohydrate count, but they're not necessary. You can find a delicious ham that contains only pork and salt.

2 large zucchini

1 teaspoon sea salt, divided

½ cup diced no-sugar-added ham

8 large eggs

½ cup full-fat coconut milk

¼ teaspoon ground black pepper

¼ teaspoon crushed red pepper

1 cup shredded Cheddar cheese

SERVES 6 (MAKES 12 EGG CUPS)	
Per Serving:	
Calories	122
Fat	9g
Protein	8g
Sodium	362mg
Fiber	0g
Carbohydrates	3g
Net Carbs	3g
Sugar	1g

1 Shred zucchini using a cheese grater or the shredding attachment of a food processor. Transfer zucchini to a strainer and sprinkle with ½ teaspoon salt. Toss to coat. Let zucchini sit for 30 minutes to let excess water drain out.

2 After 30 minutes, use a cheesecloth or a nut milk bag to squeeze out as much excess moisture as you can.

3 Preheat oven to 350°F. Spray each well of a muffin tin with coconut oil cooking spray.

4 Press equal amounts of zucchini into the bottom of each well. Put equal amounts of ham on top of zucchini.

5 Whisk together eggs, coconut milk, remaining ½ teaspoon salt, black pepper, and red pepper in a large bowl. Pour equal amounts of egg mixture into each well. Sprinkle cheese on top.

6 Bake for 20 minutes or until eggs are set and cheese is melted and bubbly. Remove from oven and allow to cool slightly. Remove from muffin tin and serve warm.

Mixed Berry Parfaits

FRESH OR FROZEN?

Many people think fresh is best, but that might not be true when it comes to produce. Fruits and vegetables start to lose nutrients as soon as they're picked. When fruits and vegetables are frozen, they're generally picked and then flash frozen immediately, which locks in the vitamins and minerals. The fresh produce that you find at your typical grocery store may have been picked weeks prior, losing important vitamins and minerals as time passes.

Frozen berries tend to release more juices when heated and mixed with sweetener, but if you prefer fresh berries or that's all you have on hand, you can replace the frozen berries with equal parts fresh.

½ cup plus two tablespoons frozen mixed berries

½ tablespoon water

½ tablespoon lemon juice

2 teaspoons granulated erythritol

2 tablespoons chia seeds

½ teaspoon ground cinnamon

1 cup unsweetened vanilla almond milk

2 teaspoons stevia-sweetened maple syrup

½ cup coconut cream, whipped

1 Combine berries, water, lemon juice, and erythritol in a small saucepan over medium-low heat. Bring to a simmer, stirring frequently and breaking up berries with a large spoon. Set aside.

2 Combine chia seeds, cinnamon, almond milk, and maple syrup in a small bowl. Pour equal amounts into two 16-ounce Mason jars or glass jars with lids and allow to sit for 30 minutes.

3 Scoop equal amounts of berry mixture on top of chia mixture. Scoop coconut cream on top. Chill for 30 minutes before serving.

Eggs Benedict

This classic dish is a simple but filling breakfast, and you'll find that homemade hollandaise sauce is surprisingly easy to make. You can up the fat content of this Eggs Benedict by adding a few slices of avocado under the eggs before drizzling with hollandaise sauce.

2 Keto English Muffins (see recipe in this chapter)

4 slices no-sugar-added Canadian bacon, cooked

4 large eggs

4 large egg yolks

1 teaspoon lemon juice

½ cup grass-fed butter, melted

½ teaspoon sea salt

SERVES 2	
Per Serving:	
Calories	122
Fat	11g
Protein	5g
Sodium	216mg
Fiber	0g
Carbohydrates	1g
Net Carbs	1g
Sugar	0g

1 Place two English muffin halves on two plates and top each half with a slice of Canadian bacon. Set aside.

2 Bring a medium saucepan of water to a boil over high heat, then reduce heat to low to bring to a simmer. Stir the water with a wooden spoon, and while the water is spinning, drop in an egg. Cook for 3 minutes, then remove with a slotted spoon and set on top of Canadian bacon.

3 Repeat with the remaining three eggs.

4 Discard most of the water used for poaching except for about 1 cup. Bring water to a simmer over medium-low heat and place a medium glass bowl on top of saucepan. Add egg yolks and lemon juice to bowl and whisk to combine.

5 Continue whisking while simultaneously slowly pouring butter into egg mixture to make the hollandaise sauce. Whisk in salt.

6 Scoop equal amounts of hollandaise sauce on top of each egg and serve immediately.

Jalapeño Popper Egg Cups

Jalapeño poppers and eggs are two keto diet staples. This recipe brings them together to form a deliciously creamy egg cup that tastes great hot or cold and is easy to take on the go.

**SERVES 6
(MAKES 12 EGG CUPS)**

Per Serving:

Calories	319
Fat	25g
Protein	21g
Sodium	873mg
Fiber	0g
Carbohydrates	2g
Net Carbs	2g
Sugar	1g

BE CAREFUL WITH PEPPERS!

You should always wear food-grade gloves when working with hot peppers, like jalapeños. It helps prevent the pepper from burning your skin, and it also ensures that none of the capsaicin in the pepper gets on your hand. The spicy compound can remain on the skin for hours, and if you forget and rub your eyes, it can be a painful reminder.

12 slices no-sugar-added bacon, cooked

10 large eggs

3 tablespoons sour cream

1 tablespoon cream cheese

1 cup shredded white Cheddar cheese

1 large jalapeño, seeded and minced

1 teaspoon onion salt

½ teaspoon ground black pepper

1 Preheat oven to 350°F. Line each well of a muffin tin with a paper liner.

2 Crumble bacon into the bottom of each well.

3 Combine remaining ingredients in a medium bowl and whisk together until incorporated. Pour equal amounts of egg mixture on top of bacon.

4 Bake for 25 minutes or until eggs set. Remove from oven and allow to cool slightly.

5 Remove from muffin tin and serve warm.

Bacon, Egg, and Cheese Stack

Who needs bread when you've got a bun made out of eggs? This Bacon, Egg, and Cheese Stack packs in protein and healthy fats to keep you full until lunchtime. You won't even miss the carbs!

2 large eggs

1 tablespoon unsweetened almond milk

¼ teaspoon sea salt

⅛ teaspoon ground black pepper

2 slices no-sugar-added bacon, cooked

¼ cup shredded pepper jack cheese

½ medium avocado, peeled, pitted, and lightly mashed

1 teaspoon The New Primal Medium Buffalo Dipping & Wing Sauce

1   Whisk together eggs, almond milk, salt, and pepper in a small bowl. Spray a 3¼" ramekin with coconut oil cooking spray and pour half of egg mixture into prepared microwave-safe ramekin.

2   Microwave for 45 seconds, check for doneness, and continue microwaving in 15-second intervals until eggs no longer appear wet. Remove egg from ramekin and place on a plate. Repeat with the rest of egg mixture.

3   Top one egg patty with bacon, cheese, and avocado, then place the other egg patty on top. Drizzle with buffalo sauce and serve immediately.

SERVES 1	
Per Serving:	
Calories	485
Fat	39g
Protein	28g
Sodium	1,296mg
Fiber	3g
Carbohydrates	9g
Net Carbs	6g
Sugar	1g

KETO-FRIENDLY BUFFALO SAUCE

Most store-bought buffalo sauces contain sweeteners that don't have a place in a keto-genic diet plan. In the days before keto and "clean eating" became popular, you used to have to make any sauces and condiments your-self if you wanted to make sure the ingredi-ents were appropriate. Now, many companies are rolling out all kinds of keto-friendly sauces and dressings. The New Primal and Tessemae's are two companies that make a wide range of condiments.

Baked Eggs Benedict

SERVES 6

Per Serving:

Calories	370
Fat	33g
Protein	17g
Sodium	540mg
Fiber	0g
Carbohydrates	2g
Net Carbs	2g
Sugar	0g

This Baked Eggs Benedict gives you all the favor of the traditional version without any fuss. If you eat dairy, you can add a little shredded Cheddar cheese to increase the fat content and bring out some salty flavor.

2 tablespoons grass-fed butter

¾ cup chopped no-sugar-added Canadian bacon

12 large eggs

½ cup unsweetened almond milk

1 teaspoon dry mustard powder

1 teaspoon granulated garlic

1 teaspoon granulated onion

¾ teaspoon sea salt, divided

¼ teaspoon ground black pepper

¼ teaspoon paprika

4 large egg yolks

1 teaspoon lemon juice

½ cup grass-fed butter, melted

1 Preheat oven to 350°F.

2 Heat 2 tablespoons butter in a medium skillet over medium heat. Add bacon and cook until it starts to brown, about 4 minutes.

3 Crumble then transfer to a medium mixing bowl. Add eggs, almond milk, mustard powder, garlic, onion, ¼ teaspoon salt, pepper, and paprika. Whisk until combined.

4 Pour egg mixture into a 9" × 13" baking dish and bake for 30 minutes or until eggs are set.

5 While eggs are cooking, bring water to a boil in a medium saucepan over high heat. Reduce heat to medium-low and bring water to a simmer. Place a medium glass bowl on top of saucepan. Add egg yolks and lemon juice to bowl and whisk to combine.

6 Continue whisking while simultaneously slowly pouring butter into egg mixture to make the hollandaise sauce. Whisk in remaining salt.

7 Remove eggs from oven and allow to cool. Cut into six pieces and drizzle hollandaise sauce on each piece.

Fluffy Almond Waffles

The psyllium husk in this recipe helps keep the waffles from falling apart and adds a small amount of fiber, which helps prevent constipation. You can leave it out if you don't have it, but your waffles might crumble slightly. Serve these with stevia-sweetened maple syrup or your favorite keto-friendly topping.

1 large egg, separated

½ cup blanched almond flour

2 tablespoons granulated erythritol

1 teaspoon psyllium husk

½ teaspoon baking powder

¼ teaspoon sea salt

2 tablespoons no-sugar-added peanut butter

2 tablespoons grass-fed butter

¼ cup plus 1 tablespoon full-fat coconut milk

½ teaspoon vanilla extract

⅛ teaspoon almond extract

1 Preheat waffle iron.

2 Place egg white in a medium mixing bowl and beat with a mixer until soft peaks form. In a separate medium bowl, combine almond flour, erythritol, psyllium husk, baking powder, and salt.

3 Combine peanut butter and butter in a small saucepan over low heat. Stir until melted and combined. Pour into dry ingredients and add egg yolk, coconut milk, vanilla extract, and almond extract. Stir until smooth.

4 Fold in egg whites and mix until just combined.

5 Pour half the batter into the waffle iron and cook for about 4 minutes or until waffle iron indicates waffle is done cooking. Repeat with remaining batter. Serve immediately.

SERVES 2

Per Serving:

Calories	450
Fat	31g
Protein	13g
Sodium	486mg
Fiber	5g
Carbohydrates	22g
Net Carbs	5g
Sugar	2g

WHAT IS PSYLLIUM HUSK?

Psyllium husk is a fiber made from the outer husks of the seeds from the psyllium plant. When used in recipes, it provides soluble fiber and acts as a binding agent to help keep things, especially baked goods, from falling apart. Although it does add to the total carbohydrates of a recipe, most of the carbohydrates come from fiber, which doesn't count toward your net carbohydrate count.

Sausage Gravy

SERVES 4	
Per Serving:	
Calories	496
Fat	51g
Protein	7g
Sodium	533mg
Fiber	1g
Carbohydrates	3g
Net Carbs	2g
Sugar	2g

This Sausage Gravy freezes really well and will keep for up to 6 months. Serve on top of Keto English Muffins (see recipe in this chapter) for a low-carb take on biscuits and gravy.

½ pound no-sugar-added pork breakfast sausage

2 tablespoons grass-fed butter

1½ cups grass-fed heavy cream

¾ teaspoon guar gum

¼ teaspoon seasoned salt

¼ teaspoon garlic powder

¼ teaspoon ground black pepper

1 Heat a medium skillet over medium-high heat. Crumble sausage into hot skillet and cook until no longer pink, about 7 minutes. Add butter to pan and stir until melted.

2 Pour in cream and guar gum and whisk constantly until mixture starts to thicken. Stir in spices. Remove from heat and serve hot.

Vanilla Almond Chia Pudding

SERVES 2	
Per Serving:	
Calories	267
Fat	21g
Protein	9g
Sodium	269mg
Fiber	13g
Carbohydrates	16g
Net Carbs	3g
Sugar	1g

If you prefer your chia seeds whole, leave them out of the food processor and then mix them in after processing.

3½ tablespoons whole chia seeds

1 tablespoon vanilla MCT oil powder

⅔ cup unsweetened vanilla almond milk

2 tablespoons no-sugar-added almond butter

1½ tablespoons stevia-sweetened maple syrup

½ teaspoon vanilla extract

⅛ teaspoon sea salt

1 Place chia seeds in food processor and process for 30 seconds until a powder is formed. Add remaining ingredients and process for 30 seconds, scrape down the bowl, and process for another 30 seconds.

2 Transfer to two 8-ounce Mason jars or any glass jars with lids and cover. Refrigerate for 1 hour before serving.

Baked Egg Spanakopita

Don't have frozen spinach? Not a problem! You can use 1 pound of fresh spinach in place of frozen in this recipe and any other that calls for it. This is a crowd-pleasing dish to bring to a potluck brunch—you'll ensure that you have a keto-friendly option to eat, and everyone else will just enjoy the rich, delicious flavors!

1 tablespoon olive oil

2 small shallots, peeled and minced

1½ teaspoons minced garlic

1 (10-ounce) package frozen chopped spinach, thawed and drained

1 (16-ounce) container full-fat cottage cheese

6 large eggs

¼ teaspoon dried dill

¼ teaspoon sea salt

½ cup crumbled feta cheese

1 Preheat oven to 350°F.

2 Heat oil in a medium skillet over medium heat. Add shallots and garlic and cook until softened, about 4 minutes. Add spinach and cook until spinach is heated through, another 2 minutes. Remove from heat and set aside.

3 Combine remaining ingredients in a large mixing bowl. Fold in spinach mixture and stir until combined.

4 Transfer into an 8" × 8" baking dish and bake for 45 minutes or until eggs are set. Remove from heat and allow to cool slightly.

5 Cut into six squares and serve warm.

SERVES 6	
Per Serving:	
Calories	224
Fat	12g
Protein	20g
Sodium	644mg
Fiber	2g
Carbohydrates	9g
Net Carbs	7g
Sugar	5g

BABY VERSUS MATURE SPINACH

Baby spinach comes from the smallest leaves of the spinach plant and is typically harvested early, around 15 to 35 days after planting. Mature spinach comes from the leaves that are allowed to grow fully. Baby spinach has a milder taste but tends to turn slimy when cooked. As a general rule, it's best to eat baby spinach raw and use mature spinach when cooking.

Keto Crepes

SERVES 2

Per Serving:

Calories	408
Fat	38g
Protein	13g
Sodium	286mg
Fiber	0g
Carbohydrates	4g
Net Carbs	4g
Sugar	2g

These crepes are excellent as part of your breakfast, or you can use them as a wrap to make your favorite keto sandwiches. Serve with your favorite keto-friendly toppings, such as stevia-sweetened maple syrup, coconut flakes, crushed walnuts, or avocado slices.

4 ounces cream cheese, softened

3 large eggs

2 tablespoons grass-fed butter

1 Combine cream cheese and eggs in a blender and blend until smooth.

2 Heat butter in a medium skillet over medium heat. Pour 2 tablespoons of batter into pan and cook for 2 minutes or until crepe starts to turn golden brown. Flip and cook for another minute. Transfer to a serving dish.

3 Repeat until all the batter is gone and serve.

Vanilla Cinnamon Overnight "Oats"

SERVES 1

Per Serving:

Calories	562
Fat	42g
Protein	30g
Sodium	423mg
Fiber	13g
Carbohydrates	25g
Net Carbs	4g
Sugar	2g

Like chia pudding, this mixture will thicken as it sits in the refrigerator. If you prefer a thinner consistency, stir in a little almond milk before serving.

⅔ cup unsweetened vanilla almond milk

½ cup hemp hearts

1 tablespoon chia seeds

2 teaspoons powdered erythritol

¾ teaspoon vanilla extract

⅛ teaspoon sea salt

½ teaspoon ground cinnamon

1 Combine all ingredients in a 16-ounce Mason jar or a glass jar with a lid. Cover and shake vigorously until combined.

2 Refrigerate overnight, or for at least 8 hours.

3 Serve cold.

CHAPTER 3

Keto Lunch

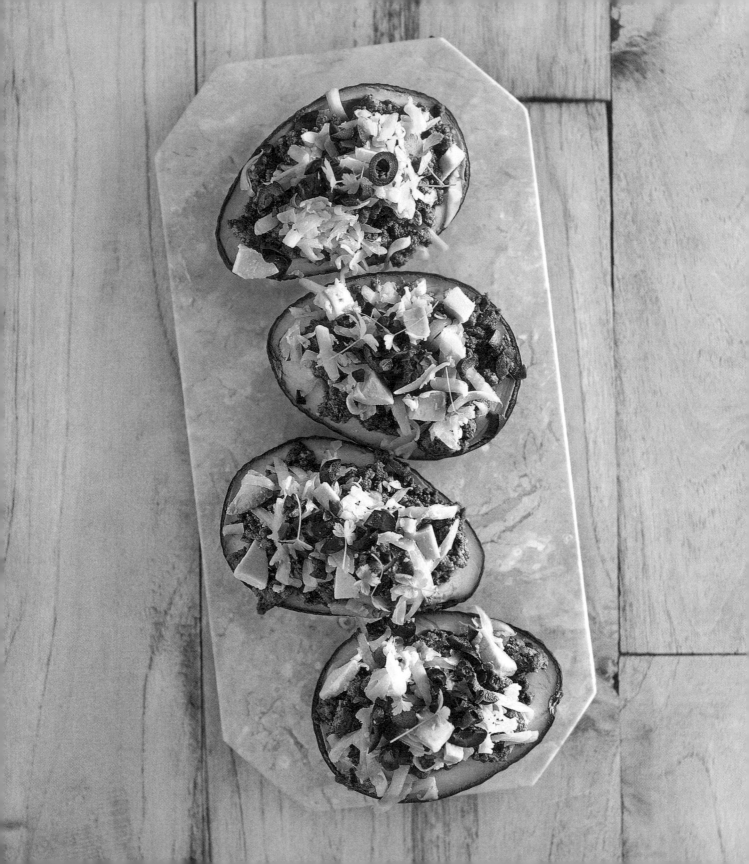

Taco-Stuffed Avocados

There's no need to skip Taco Tuesday when you're on a keto diet. Lose the tortillas in favor of an avocado half for a perfectly balanced, fat-rich meal that offers authentic taco flavors.

½ pound 85/15 ground beef

½ tablespoon chili powder

¾ teaspoon ground cumin

¼ teaspoon paprika

⅛ teaspoon dried oregano

⅛ teaspoon red pepper flakes

⅛ teaspoon granulated garlic

⅛ teaspoon granulated onion

½ teaspoon sea salt

½ teaspoon ground black pepper

2 tablespoons tomato sauce

2 medium avocados, peeled

¼ cup shredded Cheddar cheese

2 tablespoons chopped black olives

4 teaspoons chopped fresh cilantro

1   Heat a medium skillet over medium-high heat. Add ground beef and cook until no longer pink, about 7 minutes. Add spices and tomato sauce and stir until incorporated. Reduce heat to low and cook for another 3 minutes.

2   Cut avocados in half lengthwise and remove the pit. Scoop out a little well in each avocado half. Chop up avocado that you scooped out and set aside.

3   Spoon equal amounts of beef mixture into each avocado half. Top with equal amounts of cheese, olives, chopped avocado, and cilantro. Serve immediately.

SERVES 2	
Per Serving:	
Calories	529
Fat	40g
Protein	30g
Sodium	1,100mg
Fiber	7g
Carbohydrates	19g
Net Carbs	12g
Sugar	1g

CILANTRO THE CHELATOR

Cilantro does more than make your taco bowls taste delicious; it also acts as a chelating agent. In other words, compounds in cilantro react to heavy metal ions, turning them into stable water-soluble substances that your body can effectively detoxify. Why is this important? When you combine fish, like tuna, that's high in mercury, with cilantro, the cilantro helps negate the adverse effect mercury can have on your body.

BLT-Stuffed Avocados

SERVES 2

Per Serving:

Calories	509
Fat	46g
Protein	14g
Sodium	777mg
Fiber	5g
Carbohydrates	17g
Net Carbs	12g
Sugar	2g

MAKING YOUR OWN MAYO

Fortunately, several companies now make keto-friendly mayonnaises that you can find in a lot of big-name grocery stores or order online. It's also easy to make with an immersion blender. Just combine one room-temperature egg, the fresh juice from ½ a room-temperature lemon, ¾ teaspoon dry mustard powder, ½ teaspoon sea salt, and ½ teaspoon white pepper in a medium bowl. Use the immersion blender to blend everything together until an emulsion forms. Store in an airtight glass container in the refrigerator for up to 1 week.

Bacon makes everything better, and these BLT-Stuffed Avocados are no exception. The saltiness of the bacon pairs nicely with the creamy texture of the avocados, and they both provide you with the fats you need to stay in ketosis.

2 medium avocados, peeled

4 slices no-sugar-added bacon, cooked and chopped

⅓ cup chopped grape tomatoes

⅓ cup chopped romaine lettuce

2 tablespoons keto-friendly mayonnaise

1 teaspoon lime juice

¼ teaspoon sea salt

¼ teaspoon ground black pepper

1 Cut avocados in half lengthwise and remove the pit. Scoop out a little well in each avocado half. Chop up avocado that you scooped out and set aside.

2 Combine chopped avocado and remaining ingredients in a small bowl and stir until incorporated. Spoon equal amounts of bacon mixture into each avocado well. Serve immediately.

Egg Salad–Stuffed Avocados

If you're on the go or you want to make these more portable, you can scoop the avocado flesh from the avocado, mash it, and mix it into the egg salad before eating.

2 medium avocados, peeled

4 hard-boiled eggs

3 tablespoons keto-friendly mayonnaise

¼ teaspoon sea salt

¼ teaspoon ground black pepper

¼ teaspoon dry mustard powder

2 tablespoons everything bagel seasoning

1 Cut avocados in half lengthwise and remove the pit. Scoop out a little well in each avocado half. Chop up avocado that you scooped out and set aside.

2 Combine remaining ingredients, except for chopped avocado and bagel seasoning, in a medium mixing bowl and mash with a fork until incorporated. Stir in chopped avocado.

3 Scoop equal amounts of egg mixture into each avocado well. Sprinkle everything bagel seasoning on top.

SERVES 2	
Per Serving:	
Calories	603
Fat	50g
Protein	18g
Sodium	1,546mg
Fiber	5g
Carbohydrates	16g
Net Carbs	11g
Sugar	0g

THE SECRET TO THE PERFECT HARD-BOILED EGG

There's a lot of argument about how to make the perfectly cooked hard-boiled egg, but here's a foolproof way: Place eggs in a small saucepan and pour in just enough cold water to cover them. Bring them to a boil over high heat. Once they start boiling, cook them for 1 minute, then cover, remove them from the heat, and let them sit for 12 minutes. After 12 minutes, immediately submerge them in an ice bath. Once cooled, peel and use!

Ham and Turkey Roll-Ups

Make sure you read the ingredient lists when buying deli meats. Ask the deli counter staff to show you the ingredient lists before making your choices. Don't be shy!

4 slices no-sugar-added uncured ham

4 slices no-sugar-added roasted turkey

4 slices provolone cheese

2 tablespoons banana peppers

2 tablespoons keto-friendly mayonnaise

2 teaspoons yellow mustard

2 tablespoons chopped roasted red peppers

1 Layer a slice of ham, turkey, and provolone cheese four times to make four stacks. Top each stack with banana peppers, mayonnaise, mustard, and red peppers.

2 Carefully roll stacks tightly and secure the edges with toothpicks.

Greek Zoodle Mason Jar Salad

If you don't have a spiralizer, you can cube the zucchini instead.

2 tablespoons extra-virgin olive oil

2 tablespoons lemon juice

1 teaspoon dried oregano

¼ teaspoon sea salt

¼ teaspoon ground black pepper

½ cup cubed cooked chicken

¼ cup chopped peeled red onion

¼ cup chopped pitted Kalamata olives

¼ cup crumbled feta cheese

2 medium zucchini, spiralized

1 Whisk together olive oil, lemon juice, oregano, salt, and pepper in a small bowl. Put 2 tablespoons of dressing in the bottom of each of two 1-quart widemouthed Mason jars.

2 Layer ¼ cup chicken, 2 tablespoons red onion, 2 tablespoons olives, 2 tablespoons feta cheese, and half of zucchini zoodles in each jar. Store in the refrigerator for up to 1 week. Shake before serving.

Cheeseburger Salad

This Cheeseburger Salad tastes like a fast-food chain's most popular burger, but without any of the undesirable ingredients that come with it. If you're enjoying it on one of your higher-carb days, you can use relish, which adds a nice sweetness, in place of the dill pickles.

1 pound 85/15 ground beef

1 teaspoon sea salt

½ teaspoon ground black pepper

½ teaspoon granulated garlic

4 cups chopped iceberg lettuce

¼ cup chopped peeled yellow onion

¼ cup chopped cherry tomatoes

¼ cup shredded Cheddar cheese

⅛ cup chopped dill pickles

¼ cup keto-friendly mayonnaise

¼ cup no-sugar-added ketchup

¼ cup Dijon mustard

1½ tablespoons pickle juice

1 Heat a medium skillet over medium-high heat. Add ground beef and cook until no longer pink, about 7 minutes. Add salt, pepper, and garlic. Remove from heat and allow to cool completely.

2 Combine lettuce, onions, tomatoes, cheese, pickles, and cooled beef in a medium bowl and toss until incorporated.

3 In a small bowl, whisk together remaining ingredients until smooth. Pour over beef mixture and toss to fully coat. Serve immediately.

SERVES 4

Per Serving:

Calories	348
Fat	26g
Protein	23g
Sodium	1,598mg
Fiber	0g
Carbohydrates	8g
Net Carbs	8g
Sugar	2g

PICKLE JUICE: THE NATURAL SPORTS DRINK

Pickle juice contains calcium, sodium, potassium, and magnesium—four electrolytes that are lost during sweat and excessive exercise. Drinking pickle juice after periods of exercise can help replenish those electrolytes and keep you hydrated, without the sugars and artificial ingredients that are found in many popular sports drinks.

Buffalo Chicken Pepper Boats

SERVES 4	
Per Serving:	
Calories	191
Fat	7g
Protein	15g
Sodium	810mg
Fiber	1g
Carbohydrates	8g
Net Carbs	7g
Sugar	0g

If you want to make this recipe a little more budget-friendly, you can swap the orange peppers for green or red.

2 large orange bell peppers

1 (12.5-ounce) can cooked chicken breast

¼ cup The New Primal Medium Buffalo Dipping & Wing Sauce

¼ cup finely chopped celery

¼ cup Tessemae's Organic Creamy Ranch dressing

1 Cut tops off bell peppers and remove seeds. Cut each pepper in half lengthwise, then cut each half in half. Set aside.

2 Combine remaining ingredients in a medium bowl.

3 Scoop equal amounts of chicken mixture onto each piece of bell pepper. Serve immediately.

Cheesy Cauliflower and Pork Hash

SERVES 6	
Per Serving:	
Calories	252
Fat	19g
Protein	15g
Sodium	659mg
Fiber	1g
Carbohydrates	5g
Net Carbs	4g
Sugar	2g

When working with frozen riced cauliflower, you don't have to let it thaw before cooking it. You can use it right out of the freezer.

1 pound ground no-sugar-added hot Italian sausage

1 (12-ounce) bag frozen riced cauliflower

½ teaspoon sea salt

¼ teaspoon ground black pepper

1 cup shredded Cheddar cheese

1 Heat a medium skillet over medium-high heat. Crumble sausage into pan and cook until no longer pink, about 7 minutes.

2 Reduce heat to medium. Stir in cauliflower, salt, and pepper and cook until cauliflower is tender, another 4 minutes. Stir in Cheddar cheese, cover, and cook for another 2 minutes or until cheese is melted and bubbly.

3 Remove from heat, allow to cool slightly, and serve.

Salmon Cobb Mason Jar Salad

The salmon in this recipe adds a significant amount of omega-3 fatty acids to this salad. You can cook some fresh fillets instead of using canned salmon, if you prefer, or use another protein source instead; but keep in mind that doing so will change the fat content.

¼ cup Tessemae's Organic Creamy Ranch Dressing

1 (6-ounce) can wild Alaskan pink salmon

¼ cup chopped hard-boiled egg

¼ cup chopped cooked no-sugar-added bacon

¼ cup chopped, peeled, and pitted avocado

¼ cup crumbled blue cheese

¼ cup chopped grape tomatoes

2 tablespoons minced peeled red onion

2 cups chopped iceberg lettuce

1   Put 2 tablespoons of dressing in the bottom of each of two 1-quart widemouthed Mason jars.

2   Layer 3 ounces salmon, 2 tablespoons hard-boiled egg, 2 tablespoons bacon, 2 tablespoons avocado, 2 tablespoons blue cheese, 2 tablespoons tomatoes, 1 tablespoon red onion, and 1 cup lettuce in each jar.

3   Store in the refrigerator for up to 1 week. When ready to eat, shake vigorously and then serve.

SERVES 2

Per Serving:

Calories	449
Fat	26g
Protein	31g
Sodium	917mg
Fiber	2g
Carbohydrates	5g
Net Carbs	3g
Sugar	1g

GETTING YOUR OMEGA-3S

Omega-3 fatty acids are classified as essential fats because, unlike other fats, your body can't make them; you have to get them from your diet. They're highly important because they affect the function of all of your cells. Omega-3 fats play huge roles in preventing heart disease and stroke and reducing inflammation. Salmon is one of the richest sources, offering a whopping 2,260 milligrams per 3½ ounces. Most health experts recommend getting between 250 and 500 milligrams per day.

Parmesan-Coated Chicken

SERVES 4

Per Serving:

Calories	301
Fat	19g
Protein	28g
Sodium	816mg
Fiber	1g
Carbohydrates	4g
Net Carbs	3g
Sugar	0g

The Parmesan coating in this recipe is great on chicken as well as white fish. Switching up your protein sources can easily create variety for busy weeknight meals that use simple ingredients.

¼ **cup paleo flour**

½ **cup grated Parmesan cheese**

1 teaspoon paprika

½ **teaspoon dried parsley**

½ **teaspoon garlic powder**

1 teaspoon sea salt

½ **teaspoon ground black pepper**

4 (4-ounce) boneless, skinless chicken breasts

1 large egg, lightly beaten

¼ **cup grass-fed butter, melted**

1 Preheat oven to 350°F.

2 Combine paleo flour, Parmesan cheese, paprika, parsley, garlic powder, salt, and pepper in a medium shallow bowl. Mix until incorporated.

3 Dip each chicken breast into egg and then place in flour mixture, tossing to coat completely.

4 Arrange chicken in a 9" × 13" baking dish and pour melted butter over chicken breasts.

5 Bake for 45 minutes or until chicken is no longer pink and juices run clear.

6 Remove from oven, allow to cool slightly, and serve.

Baked Stuffed Avocados

When broiling these avocados, watch them closely! Cheese can burn quickly under the broiler, especially if the rack is positioned really closely to the top of the oven.

2 medium avocados, peeled, pitted, and cut in half lengthwise

2 (4-ounce) chicken breasts, cooked and shredded

2 ounces cream cheese, softened

¼ teaspoon sea salt

¼ teaspoon ground black pepper

¼ teaspoon garlic powder

⅛ teaspoon cayenne pepper

2 tablespoons chopped fresh cilantro

⅛ cup shredded Parmesan cheese

⅛ cup shredded Cheddar cheese

1   Preheat oven to 400°F.

2   Scoop out a little bit of avocado from each half and roughly chop. Transfer to a medium bowl.

3   Add chicken, cream cheese, salt, pepper, garlic powder, cayenne pepper, and cilantro and mix to combine.

4   Scoop equal amounts of chicken mixture into each avocado half. Arrange stuffed avocados in an 8" × 8" baking dish and bake for 10 minutes.

5   Turn oven to broil. Sprinkle cheeses on top and broil for 4 minutes or until cheese is melted and bubbly.

6   Remove from oven, allow to cool slightly, and serve.

SERVES 2	
Per Serving:	
Calories	532
Fat	40g
Protein	33g
Sodium	593mg
Fiber	5g
Carbohydrates	18g
Net Carbs	13g
Sugar	1g

CHOOSING A PERFECTLY RIPE AVOCADO

There's nothing that brings happiness to a keto dieter quite like the perfectly ripe avocado. You can choose one every time by looking for two things—consistency and color. An avocado that's ready to eat feels firm but gives a little bit to slight pressure. You shouldn't see any indentations or feel mushiness. Although color can vary, a dark green to black color usually indicates that the avocado is ripe.

Garlic Lime Chicken

SERVES 4

Per Serving:

Calories	108
Fat	4g
Protein	16g
Sodium	597mg
Fiber	0g
Carbohydrates	2g
Net Carbs	2g
Sugar	0g

Although you can buy bottled lime juice, nothing quite gives the same flavor as the juice from a fresh lime, so try to squeeze your own juice for this recipe. You can buy a manual citrus squeezer for under $20 at most home stores if you want to be sure to get the maximum amount of juice out of fruits.

1 teaspoon sea salt

½ teaspoon ground black pepper

¼ teaspoon cayenne pepper

¼ teaspoon paprika

½ teaspoon garlic powder

½ teaspoon onion powder

½ teaspoon dried parsley

4 (4-ounce) boneless, skinless chicken thighs

¼ cup fresh lime juice

1 Preheat oven to 350°F.

2 Combine salt, black pepper, cayenne pepper, paprika, garlic powder, onion powder, and parsley in a small bowl and stir until incorporated.

3 Arrange chicken thighs in a 9" × 13" baking dish and sprinkle spice mixture over chicken, coating as much of each thigh as possible. Bake for 25 minutes.

4 Sprinkle lime juice over chicken thighs and cook for an additional 20 minutes or until chicken is no longer pink and juices run clear.

5 Remove from oven, allow to cool slightly, and serve.

Juicy Turkey Burgers

Although these Juicy Turkey Burgers are lower in fat than their ground beef counterparts, there's no flavor lost. You can add some healthy fats to the recipe by topping the finished burgers with cheese (if you eat it), sliced avocado, and some keto-friendly ranch dressing. Then serve with your favorite vegetable side dish.

1 pound ground turkey

1 tablespoon coarse almond meal

1 teaspoon dried parsley

1 tablespoon dried minced onion

1 large egg, lightly beaten

1 teaspoon minced garlic

½ teaspoon sea salt

¼ teaspoon ground black pepper

½ teaspoon coconut aminos

1 Combine all ingredients in a large bowl and mix until incorporated. Form mixture into four equal-sized patties.

2 Heat a medium skillet or griddle over medium heat. Arrange patties on hot skillet and cook for 4 minutes. Flip and cook for an additional 4 minutes or until turkey is no longer pink.

3 Remove from heat and serve.

SERVES 4	
Per Serving:	
Calories	192
Fat	10g
Protein	23g
Sodium	348mg
Fiber	0g
Carbohydrates	2g
Net Carbs	2g
Sugar	1g

COCONUT WHAT-OS?

Coconut aminos is a sauce made from coconut sap. Its flavor is similar to that of a light soy sauce or tamari, but without the soy. In addition to being soy-free, coconut aminos is gluten free and paleo-friendly, and it contains all of the nine essential amino acids. It's a great addition to your keto cabinet for any time you need to add that umami flavor to one of your recipes.

Creamy Stuffed Chicken Breasts

SERVES 4

Per Serving:

Calories	308
Fat	20g
Protein	29g
Sodium	845mg
Fiber	0g
Carbohydrates	2g
Net Carbs	2g
Sugar	1g

These Creamy Stuffed Chicken Breasts aren't overly hot, but if you want to dial down the spice to suit your taste, you can replace the pepper jack cheese with your favorite milder cheese. Mozzarella, Cheddar, and Monterey jack all work well.

4 (4-ounce) boneless, skinless chicken breasts

1 teaspoon seasoning salt, divided

4 ounces cream cheese, softened

¼ cup shredded pepper jack cheese

1 teaspoon minced garlic

2 tablespoons chopped green onion

¼ teaspoon sea salt

¼ teaspoon ground black pepper

8 slices no-sugar-added bacon

1 Preheat oven to 400°F.

2 Pound chicken breasts to ½" thickness. Sprinkle ½ teaspoon of seasoning salt over chicken breasts.

3 Combine cream cheese, pepper jack cheese, garlic, green onion, salt, and pepper in a small bowl. Stir until incorporated.

4 Scoop equal amounts of mixture onto each chicken breast and spread evenly with a spoon. Roll chicken breasts and secure with a toothpick. Sprinkle remaining seasoning salt on top of breasts.

5 Wrap two slices of bacon around each breast, using toothpicks to secure in place.

6 Arrange chicken breasts in a 9" × 13" baking dish and bake for 40 minutes.

7 Turn oven to broil and cook for 2 minutes, flip, and cook for another 2 minutes or until bacon starts to crisp.

8 Remove from oven, remove toothpicks, and serve.

Spinach and Feta Turkey Burgers

Make sure the frozen spinach is squeezed dry before mixing it with the other ingredients in this recipe. It will prevent the burgers from getting soggy and help make sure they stay together. Use a cheesecloth or a nut milk bag to get all of the excess moisture out.

1 pound ground turkey

1 large egg, lightly beaten

1 teaspoon minced garlic

¼ cup crumbled feta cheese

1 (10-ounce) package frozen chopped spinach, thawed and squeezed dry

½ teaspoon sea salt

¼ teaspoon ground black pepper

1 teaspoon coconut aminos

2 tablespoons avocado oil

1 Combine all ingredients, except avocado oil, in a medium bowl and mix until just incorporated.

2 Form mixture into four equal-sized patties.

3 Heat avocado oil in a medium skillet over medium-high heat. Cook patties for 4 minutes, flip, and cook for an additional 4 minutes or until turkey is no longer pink.

4 Remove from heat and serve.

SERVES 4

Per Serving:

Calories	245
Fat	16g
Protein	23g
Sodium	547mg
Fiber	2g
Carbohydrates	4g
Net Carbs	2g
Sugar	1g

CONSIDERING THE SMOKE POINT

Smoke point refers to the temperature at which an oil starts to burn and create smoke. Different types of oils have different smoke points, and because of that, they're suitable for different types of cooking. Avocado oil has a high smoke point, making it an ideal choice for high-heat cooking. Olive oil's smoke point is lower, so it's more suitable for low-heat cooking.

Buffalo Chicken Mason Jar Salad

SERVES 2	
Per Serving:	
Calories	461
Fat	26g
Protein	28g
Sodium	1,625mg
Fiber	3g
Carbohydrates	10g
Net Carbs	7g
Sugar	2g

Ranch dressing, hard-boiled eggs, black olives, and avocado all add healthy fats to this spicy Buffalo Chicken Mason Jar Salad that's easy to prepare in advance and take with you to work.

2 (4.5-ounce) cans cooked chicken breast

¼ cup The New Primal Medium Buffalo Dipping & Wing Sauce

¼ cup Tessemae's Organic Creamy Ranch Dressing

2 large hard-boiled eggs, roughly chopped

2 tablespoons minced seeded green bell pepper

2 tablespoons minced cucumber

¼ cup chopped black olives

½ cup chopped avocado

2 cups chopped romaine lettuce

1 Combine chicken breast and buffalo sauce in a medium bowl and toss to coat.

2 Scoop 2 tablespoons of ranch dressing into the bottom of two 1-quart widemouthed Mason jars and layer equal parts chicken, one chopped egg, 1 tablespoon bell pepper, 1 tablespoon cucumber, 2 tablespoons black olives, ¼ cup avocado, and 1 cup lettuce on top.

3 Cover and store in the refrigerator for up to 1 week. When ready to eat, shake vigorously before serving.

Lemon Salmon Burgers

These burgers call for canned salmon, but make sure it's the wild Alaskan salmon. Wild-caught fish is significantly more nutritious and less contaminated than farm-raised fish.

3 (6-ounce) cans wild Alaskan salmon

2 large eggs, lightly beaten

¼ cup chopped fresh parsley

2 tablespoons minced peeled white onion

¼ cup coarse almond meal

½ teaspoon Italian seasoning

2 tablespoons lemon juice

¼ teaspoon sea salt

¼ teaspoon ground black pepper

⅛ teaspoon crushed red pepper

½ cup Tessemae's Organic Habanero Ranch Dressing

1 Preheat oven to 325°F. Line a baking sheet with parchment paper.

2 Combine all ingredients, except ranch dressing, in a medium bowl and mix until just incorporated. Form into four equal-sized patties and arrange patties on prepared baking sheet.

3 Bake for 10 minutes, flip burgers over, and then bake for an additional 10 minutes.

4 Serve each burger with 2 tablespoons of ranch dressing.

SERVES 4

Per Serving:

Calories	459
Fat	26g
Protein	31g
Sodium	822mg
Fiber	1g
Carbohydrates	4g
Net Carbs	3g
Sugar	1g

GO WILD

Wild-caught fish is not only more nutritious than its farmed-raised counterparts, but it also contains significantly fewer toxins. According to reports, farm-raised salmon contains almost ten times as many PCBs (polychlorinated biphenyls), a toxin that increases the risk of stroke, insulin resistance, obesity, and diabetes. It's also higher in dioxins, a toxin that's been linked to heart disease, infertility, and hormonal issues.

Ranch Chicken with Roasted Vegetables

SERVES 4

Per Serving:

Calories	201
Fat	7g
Protein	28g
Sodium	1,206mg
Fiber	1g
Carbohydrates	5g
Net Carbs	4g
Sugar	1g

You can whip up this one-pan meal in minutes, making it perfect for a quick lunch now or for weekly meal prep. To increase the variety of vitamins and minerals, you can add in any keto-friendly vegetables you want with the broccoli and cauliflower. The ranch herbs and buffalo sauce are a classic combination.

½ teaspoon dried parsley

½ teaspoon dried dill

½ teaspoon dried chives

½ teaspoon granulated garlic

½ teaspoon granulated onion

½ teaspoon sea salt

¼ teaspoon ground black pepper

4 (4-ounce) boneless, skinless chicken breasts

1 cup chopped cauliflower florets

1 cup chopped broccoli florets

4 slices no-sugar-added bacon, cooked and roughly chopped

2 tablespoons butter-flavored coconut oil, melted

¼ cup The New Primal buffalo sauce

1 Preheat oven to 400°F. Line a baking sheet with parchment paper.

2 Combine parsley, dill, chives, garlic, onion, salt, and pepper in a small bowl. Mix until incorporated.

3 Arrange chicken, cauliflower, and broccoli in a single layer on prepared baking sheet. Sprinkle spice mixture and chopped bacon on top. Drizzle with coconut oil.

4 Bake for 20 minutes, flip vegetables and chicken, and bake for another 20 minutes or until chicken is no longer pink and juices run clear.

5 Remove from oven and drizzle buffalo sauce on top. Serve warm.

Five-Minute Creamy Tomato Soup

This soup comes together in just minutes, with ingredients that you likely already have on hand. It's great for when you need lunch in a pinch, and it goes perfectly alongside warm Keto English Muffins (see recipe in Chapter 2). Double or triple the batch so you can use it as an easy snack or freeze it for later.

1 (15-ounce) can tomato sauce

1 (8-ounce) can tomato sauce

1 cup grass-fed half-and-half

1½ teaspoons golden monk fruit sweetener

1 teaspoon Italian seasoning

½ teaspoon dried basil

½ teaspoon dried parsley

½ teaspoon sea salt

¼ teaspoon ground black pepper

½ teaspoon Frank's RedHot Original Cayenne Pepper Sauce

3 tablespoons shredded Parmesan cheese

1 Combine all ingredients, except Parmesan cheese, in a medium saucepan over medium heat. Whisk frequently until heated through, about 5 minutes.

2 Stir in Parmesan cheese.

3 Remove from heat and serve.

SERVES 2	
Per Serving:	
Calories	266
Fat	16g
Protein	11g
Sodium	2,337mg
Fiber	5g
Carbohydrates	24g
Net Carbs	16g
Sugar	17g

YOUR OWN ITALIAN BLEND

Italian seasoning is a blend of the most commonly used Italian spices, like basil, oregano, rosemary, and thyme. You can make your own by combining 1 tablespoon each dried basil, dried oregano, dried rosemary, dried marjoram, dried cilantro, and dried thyme. If you want a little kick, add 1 to 3 teaspoons of crushed red pepper too. Use what you need and store the rest in an airtight container in your spice cabinet for up to 6 months.

Grilled Bison Burgers

Bison is leaner than beef, so watch these burgers closely as they're cooking. If you cook them for too long, they can dry out quickly.

BISON OR BEEF?

Choosing a leaner beef isn't always the goal on a keto diet, but it offers some other desirable health benefits. Bison are typically raised on ranches or farms, unlike conventional cattle, which are often raised in high-production operations. Regulations prevent the use of hormones and antibiotics in bison, while they are often given to cattle to make them grow faster. Because bison are usually grass-fed, bison meat is also higher in omega-3 fats than beef from cattle that have been grain-fed.

1 pound ground bison

¼ cup almond meal

1 large egg

1 tablespoon coconut aminos

½ teaspoon Frank's RedHot Original Cayenne Pepper Sauce

½ teaspoon granulated garlic

1 teaspoon dried minced onion

½ teaspoon sea salt

¼ teaspoon ground black pepper

2 tablespoons avocado oil

1 Combine bison, almond meal, egg, coconut aminos, hot sauce, garlic, onion, salt, and pepper in a medium bowl and mix until incorporated.

2 Form mixture into four patties.

3 Heat avocado oil in a medium skillet over medium-high heat. Cook burgers for 3 minutes, flip, and cook for an additional 3 minutes or until no longer pink.

4 Remove from heat and serve.

BLT Chicken Mason Jar Salad

If you're meal prepping, you can double or triple this recipe and store the salads in your refrigerator for up to a week. The vegetables stay crisp because you don't mix the dressing with them until right before you're ready to eat.

4 tablespoons keto-friendly mayonnaise

½ teaspoon lemon juice

1 teaspoon minced green onion

⅛ teaspoon sea salt

⅛ teaspoon ground black pepper

½ cup chopped cooked no-sugar-added bacon

1 cup chopped cooked chicken

1 cup chopped Roma tomato

½ cup chopped avocado

2 cups chopped romaine lettuce

SERVES 2	
Per Serving:	
Calories	536
Fat	42g
Protein	33g
Sodium	898mg
Fiber	4g
Carbohydrates	10g
Net Carbs	6g
Sugar	4g

1 Combine mayonnaise, lemon juice, green onion, salt, and pepper in a small bowl and whisk until smooth. Scoop 2 tablespoons of dressing into the bottom of each of two 1-quart widemouthed Mason jars.

2 Layer ¼ cup bacon, ½ cup chicken, ½ cup tomato, ¼ cup avocado, and 1 cup lettuce in each jar. Cover and refrigerate for up to 1 week.

3 When ready to eat, shake vigorously and serve.

Caprese Chicken

SERVES 4

Per Serving:

Calories	315
Fat	23g
Protein	25g
Sodium	524mg
Fiber	1g
Carbohydrates	5g
Net Carbs	4g
Sugar	3g

It's best to use fresh mozzarella for this recipe rather than the slices you can find prepackaged at the grocery store. The fresh mozzarella melts better and has a richer, creamier flavor.

4 (4-ounce) boneless, skinless chicken breasts

¾ cup Primal Kitchen Italian Vinaigrette & Marinade

2 teaspoons Italian seasoning

2 teaspoons McCormick Grill Mates Montreal Chicken Seasoning

1 large beefsteak tomato, cut into 8 slices

4 slices mozzarella cheese

¼ cup chopped fresh basil leaves

1 Combine chicken, Italian vinaigrette, Italian seasoning, and Montreal chicken seasoning in a resealable plastic bag. Seal and shake vigorously to combine and coat chicken with marinade.

2 Refrigerate for 6 hours.

3 Preheat oven to 350°F.

4 Arrange marinated chicken breasts in a 9" × 13" baking dish.

5 Bake for 30 minutes. Remove chicken from oven. Top each breast with two slices of tomato and one slice of mozzarella cheese. Return to oven and bake for an additional 5 minutes or until cheese is melted.

6 Remove from oven and sprinkle fresh basil on top.

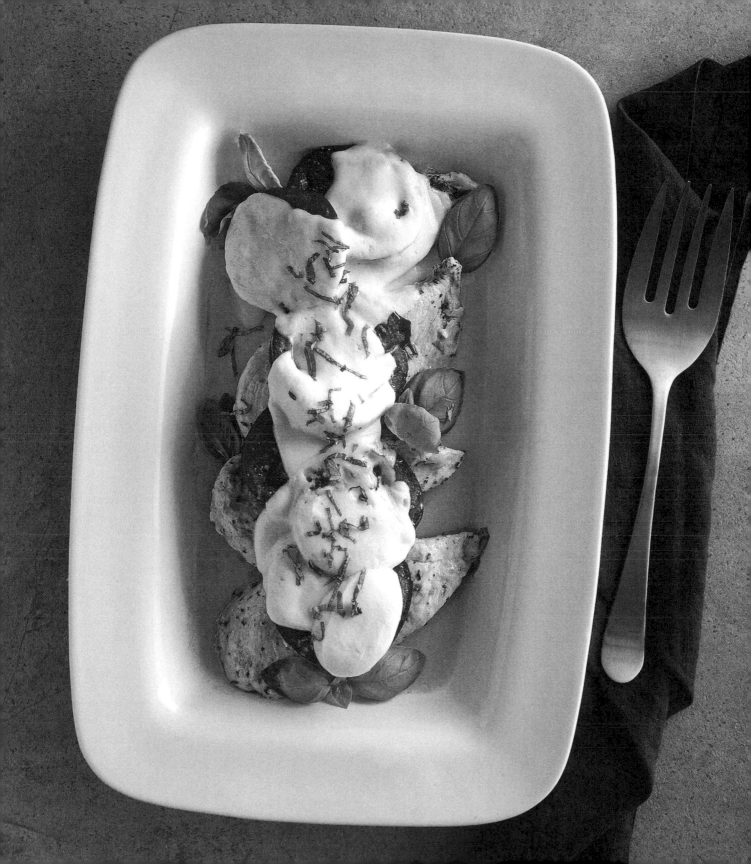

Reuben Turkey Burgers

If you love Reuben sandwiches, you'll go nuts for these Reuben Turkey Burgers. They're delicious as is, but if you want a true burger feel, you can whip up some Keto English Muffins (see recipe in Chapter 2) to use as buns.

1 pound ground turkey
1 teaspoon minced garlic
¼ cup Homemade Thousand Island Dressing
½ cup coarse almond meal
1 teaspoon Italian seasoning
½ teaspoon garlic salt
1 large egg
2 tablespoons avocado oil
4 slices Swiss cheese

1 Combine ground turkey, garlic, dressing, almond meal, seasoning, garlic salt, and egg in a medium bowl and mix until just incorporated. Shape into four equal-sized patties.

2 Heat avocado oil in a medium skillet over medium-high heat. Cook for 5 minutes, flip, and then cook for an additional 5 minutes or until turkey is no longer pink.

3 Top each patty with a slice of Swiss cheese, cover skillet, and cook for an additional 2 minutes or until cheese is melted.

4 Remove from heat and serve.

SERVES 4

Per Serving:

Calories	420
Fat	34g
Protein	29g
Sodium	577mg
Fiber	1g
Carbohydrates	6g
Net Carbs	5g
Sugar	2g

HOMEMADE THOUSAND ISLAND DRESSING

Thousand Island dressing is usually full of sugar and other artificial ingredients. Fortunately, it's easy to make at home with ingredients you likely have on hand. To make the dressing, combine ½ cup keto-friendly mayonnaise, ¼ cup keto-friendly ketchup, 2 tablespoons sweet relish, ¼ teaspoon sea salt, and ¼ teaspoon ground black pepper in a small bowl. Whisk until smooth. Use what you need and store the rest in a sealed glass jar in the refrigerator for 1 week.

Lemon Garlic Mason Jar Salad

If you don't feel like cooking your own chicken for this salad, you can use canned cooked chicken breast or buy a precooked rotisserie chicken and use the meat from that. If you use rotisserie chicken, make sure to read the ingredient list. Some of them contain added sugars.

4 tablespoons Tessemae's Organic Lemon Garlic Dressing & Marinade

½ cup shredded cooked chicken breast

¼ cup chopped cucumber

½ cup chopped cherry tomatoes

¼ cup crumbled feta cheese

¼ cup chopped hard-boiled egg

¼ cup chopped avocado

⅛ cup chopped fresh cilantro

2 cups chopped romaine lettuce

SERVES 2	
Per Serving:	
Calories	267
Fat	10g
Protein	19g
Sodium	380mg
Fiber	3g
Carbohydrates	10g
Net Carbs	7g
Sugar	3g

1 Put 2 tablespoons of dressing in the bottom of each of two 1-quart widemouthed Mason jars.

2 Scoop ¼ cup of chicken on top of dressing.

3 Layer each jar with 2 tablespoons cucumber, ¼ cup tomatoes, 2 tablespoons feta cheese, 2 tablespoons egg, 2 tablespoons avocado, 1 tablespoon cilantro, and 1 cup lettuce.

4 Cover and store in the refrigerator for up to 1 week, until ready to eat.

5 When ready to eat, shake vigorously and serve immediately.

Creamy Artichoke Soup

This Creamy Artichoke Soup has a deep, rich, salty flavor that pairs really nicely with the sage. If you want to add more vegetables, you can stir in some chopped spinach after puréeing the soup and stir it until it wilts.

¼ **cup grass-fed butter**

½ **cup chopped celery**

2 **teaspoons minced garlic**

¾ **cup chopped peeled yellow onion**

½ **cup sliced white mushrooms**

2 **tablespoons arrowroot powder**

2½ **cups chicken bone broth**

3 **(12-ounce) jars quartered artichoke hearts, drained**

½ **teaspoon sea salt**

½ **teaspoon ground black pepper**

½ **teaspoon Italian seasoning**

¼ **teaspoon dried sage**

⅛ **teaspoon paprika**

1 **cup grass-fed half-and-half**

1 Heat butter in a large stockpot over medium heat. Add celery, garlic, onion, and mushrooms and cook until softened, about 5 minutes.

2 Add arrowroot powder and stir to incorporate. Cook for 5 more minutes, stirring occasionally.

3 Add remaining ingredients, except half-and-half, and stir to combine. Reduce heat to low and simmer for 1 hour.

4 Stir in half-and-half and simmer until heated through.

5 Use an immersion blender to purée soup until smooth.

6 Remove from heat and serve.

Pesto Shrimp

This Pesto Shrimp is delicious on its own, but you can also put it on top of your favorite keto-friendly pasta substitute, like zucchini noodles, spaghetti squash, or shirataki noodles. If you'd rather have a lighter meal, try it over a salad or cauliflower rice.

¼ cup grass-fed butter

½ cup chopped seeded green bell pepper

1 cup grass-fed half-and-half

½ teaspoon ground black pepper

½ cup grated Parmesan cheese

½ cup keto-friendly pesto

1 pound raw large shrimp, peeled and deveined

¼ cup chopped fresh basil

1 Heat butter in a medium skillet over medium heat. Add peppers and cook until slightly softened, about 5 minutes. Add half-and-half and black pepper and continue cooking for 5 minutes, stirring occasionally.

2 Reduce heat to low and stir in Parmesan cheese and pesto. Cook for 5 minutes, stirring occasionally, until thickened.

3 Stir in shrimp and cook for 5 minutes or until pink. Remove from heat and stir in basil. Serve hot.

SERVES 4	
Per Serving:	
Calories	454
Fat	36g
Protein	26g
Sodium	1,239mg
Fiber	1g
Carbohydrates	6g
Net Carbs	5g
Sugar	3g

EASY HOMEMADE PESTO

You can buy a keto-friendly premade pesto at most grocery stores, but if you're having trouble finding one with ingredients that fit into your keto lifestyle, you can easily whip one up at home with a few simple ingredients. All you have to do is combine 2 cups of fresh basil, 2 cloves of garlic, ⅓ cup pine nuts, ½ cup shredded Parmesan cheese, ¼ teaspoon salt, ¼ teaspoon black pepper, and ½ cup olive oil in a food processor and process until smooth.

Beef-Fried Cauliflower Rice

SERVES 4

Per Serving:

Calories	282
Fat	16g
Protein	23g
Sodium	1,153mg
Fiber	3g
Carbohydrates	10g
Net Carbs	7g
Sugar	6g

CARBOHYDRATES IN CARROTS

Many people think carrots are completely out for a keto diet because they're known for being a higher-carb vegetable, but that's not necessarily true. One small carrot, which is equivalent to about ¼ cup chopped, contains about 6 grams of carbohydrates, 2.8 of which come from fiber. If you're watching your carbohydrates and sticking to your plan, a small amount of carrots here and there won't throw you out of ketosis.

If the carrots add too many carbohydrates for your strict keto days, you can omit them completely. On your higher-carb days, double them up to add an extra touch of crunchy sweetness.

1 tablespoon avocado oil

2 teaspoons minced garlic

½ cup diced seeded red bell pepper

½ cup diced seeded yellow bell pepper

¼ cup chopped peeled carrots

1 pound 85/15 ground beef

1 teaspoon sea salt

½ teaspoon ground black pepper

1 teaspoon freshly grated ginger

1 (12-ounce) bag frozen riced cauliflower

¼ cup coconut aminos

2 tablespoons minced green onion

1 Heat avocado oil in a medium skillet over medium heat. Add garlic and cook for 1 minute. Add bell peppers and carrots and cook until softened, about 6 minutes. Add beef, salt, and black pepper and cook until beef is no longer pink, about 7 minutes.

2 Add ginger, cauliflower, and coconut aminos and continue cooking until cauliflower softens, about 5 minutes. Stir in green onion.

3 Remove from heat and serve.

CHAPTER 4

Keto Dinner

Spaghetti Squash Pizza Bake

HOMEMADE HOT ITALIAN SAUSAGE

It's difficult to find keto-friendly hot Italian sausage at conventional grocery stores since most of them have added sweeteners, but luckily, it's easy to make your own at home. Combine 1 teaspoon sea salt, 1 teaspoon crushed fennel seeds, ¾ teaspoon crushed red pepper, 1 tablespoon paprika, and 1 teaspoon granulated garlic. Mix spices with a pound of pork, and you have fresh Italian sausage ready to go!

This is a basic recipe that you can make your own by adding any of your favorite pizza toppings. Black olives, mushrooms, green peppers, and no-sugar-added, nitrate-free pepperoni are all great keto-friendly choices.

1 pound 85/15 ground beef

½ pound no-sugar-added ground hot Italian sausage

1½ cups no-sugar-added pizza sauce

½ teaspoon dried Italian seasoning

1 medium spaghetti squash, cooked and strands and seeds removed

2 large eggs, lightly beaten

2 cups shredded mozzarella cheese

¼ cup grated Parmesan cheese

1 Preheat oven to 350°F.

2 Heat a large skillet over medium-high heat. Add ground beef and sausage and cook until no longer pink, about 7 minutes.

3 Reduce heat to medium and stir in pizza sauce and Italian seasoning. Add spaghetti squash and stir until incorporated and heated through, about 2 minutes.

4 Transfer mixture to a 9" × 13" baking dish. Stir in eggs and sprinkle both cheeses on top.

5 Bake for 45 minutes or until hot and bubbly. Remove from oven and allow to cool slightly before serving.

Decadent Crab Cakes

Crab cakes sound really fancy, but they come together in a matter of minutes. Serve them on top of a salad or with your favorite side to make them a complete meal.

2 (6-ounce) cans wild-caught crab, drained

2 tablespoons keto-friendly mayonnaise

2 large eggs

¼ cup minced seeded red bell pepper

½ cup coarse almond flour

2 tablespoons lime juice

1 teaspoon sea salt

3 tablespoons chopped fresh parsley

2 teaspoons Frank's RedHot Original Cayenne Pepper Sauce

2 tablespoons avocado oil

SERVES 2	
Per Serving:	
Calories	629
Fat	47g
Protein	44g
Sodium	2,356mg
Fiber	4g
Carbohydrates	8g
Net Carbs	4g
Sugar	2g

1 Combine all ingredients except avocado oil in a medium bowl and mix until combined.

2 Form into four equal-sized patties.

3 Heat avocado oil in a medium skillet over medium-high heat. Cook for 3 minutes, flip over, and cook for an additional 3 minutes or until golden brown.

4 Remove from heat and serve.

Taco Pie

SERVES 6

Per Serving:

Calories	295
Fat	23g
Protein	17g
Sodium	688mg
Fiber	1g
Carbohydrates	5g
Net Carbs	4g
Sugar	2g

MELTING MEXICAN BLEND

The four cheeses in Mexican blend cheese are used for their flavors and the fact that they melt quickly and easily. Most Mexican blend cheeses contain a mixture of Cheddar, Monterey jack, asadero, and queso quesadilla cheeses. If you don't have Mexican blend cheese on hand or you want to shred your own cheese, you can use any combination (or any one) of these four cheeses in any recipe that calls for it.

This Taco Pie gives you all the #tacotuesday vibes without the carbs! Top it with your favorite keto-friendly taco toppings—like sour cream, black olives, and avocado.

1 tablespoon chili powder

1½ teaspoons ground cumin

½ teaspoon paprika

1 teaspoon sea salt

1 teaspoon ground black pepper

¼ teaspoon dried oregano

¼ teaspoon crushed red pepper

¼ teaspoon granulated garlic

¼ teaspoon granulated onion

1 pound 85/15 ground beef

⅓ cup water

¼ cup finely chopped seeded green bell pepper

6 large eggs

¾ cup grass-fed half-and-half

2 ounces cream cheese

1 teaspoon minced garlic

1 cup shredded Cheddar cheese

1 cup shredded Mexican blend cheese

1 Preheat oven to 350°F.

2 Combine spices in a small bowl and stir to mix. Set aside.

3 Heat a medium skillet over medium-high heat. Crumble beef into hot pan and cook until no longer pink, about 7 minutes. Stir in spices and water and bring to a boil. Reduce heat to low and cook for 3 minutes or until mixture thickens.

4 Transfer beef to a 9" pie plate and spread in an even layer.

5 Beat green peppers, eggs, half-and-half, cream cheese, and garlic together in a medium bowl until smooth. Pour over beef mixture.

6 Sprinkle shredded cheeses on top.

7 Bake for 30 minutes or until set and cheese starts to turn golden brown.

8 Remove from oven and allow to cool slightly before serving.

Herbed Salmon Burgers

A squeeze of fresh lemon juice and a topping of tartar sauce completes these Herbed Salmon Burgers nicely.

2 (6-ounce) cans wild pink salmon

2 tablespoons chopped fresh chives

¼ cup chopped fresh parsley

¼ cup grated Parmesan cheese

2 large eggs

½ teaspoon sea salt

¼ teaspoon ground black pepper

⅓ cup coarse almond flour

2 tablespoons avocado oil

SERVES 4	
Per Serving:	
Calories	498
Fat	44g
Protein	26g
Sodium	1,246mg
Fiber	1g
Carbohydrates	2g
Net Carbs	1g
Sugar	1g

1 Combine salmon, chives, parsley, cheese, eggs, salt, and pepper in a medium bowl. Divide into four portions and form into balls. Roll each ball in almond flour and carefully flatten into patties.

2 Heat avocado oil in a medium skillet over medium heat. Cook patties for 3 minutes per side or until golden brown.

Baked Mustard Salmon

If you're not a big fan of salmon, you can re-create this recipe using any of your favorite fish. The combination of flavors works nicely with white fish as well.

4 (4-ounce) salmon fillets

⅓ cup Dijon mustard

2 teaspoons minced garlic

1 teaspoon herbes de Provence

½ teaspoon sea salt

¼ teaspoon ground black pepper

⅛ teaspoon crushed red pepper

SERVES 4	
Per Serving:	
Calories	204
Fat	11g
Protein	19g
Sodium	849mg
Fiber	0g
Carbohydrates	0g
Net Carbs	0g
Sugar	0g

1 Preheat oven to 400°F. Line a baking sheet with parchment paper.

2 Arrange salmon, skin side down, on prepared baking dish. Combine remaining ingredients in a medium bowl and spread on each salmon fillet.

3 Bake for 20 minutes or until fish flakes easily with a fork. Remove from oven and serve.

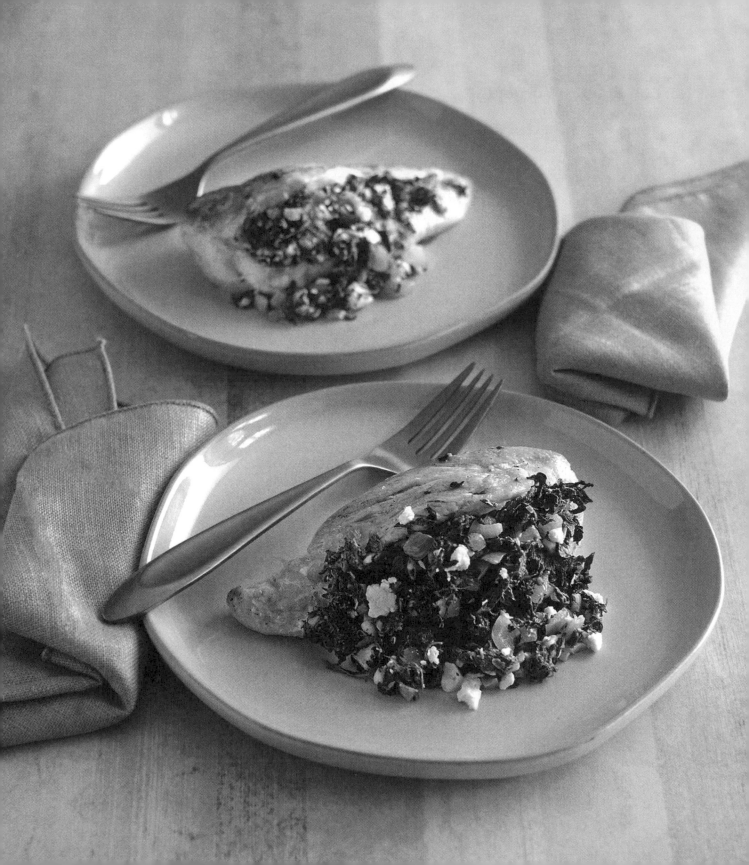

Spinach and Feta–Stuffed Chicken Breasts

This filling dish is packed with spinach, which provides folate, potassium, and vitamin C. If you have a little extra filling left over after stuffing your chicken breasts, don't throw it out! The spinach and feta mixture makes a great filling for an omelet in the morning.

2 tablespoons olive oil

2 teaspoons minced garlic

1 small yellow onion, peeled and chopped

1 (10-ounce) bag frozen chopped spinach, drained and thawed

½ teaspoon sea salt

½ teaspoon ground black pepper

¼ teaspoon crushed red pepper

⅔ cup crumbled feta cheese

4 (4-ounce) boneless, skinless chicken breasts

SERVES 4	
Per Serving:	
Calories	284
Fat	13g
Protein	30g
Sodium	951mg
Fiber	3g
Carbohydrates	7g
Net Carbs	4g
Sugar	2g

1 Preheat oven to 350°F.

2 Heat olive oil in a medium skillet over medium heat. Add garlic and onions and cook for 1 minute. Stir in spinach, salt, black pepper, and red pepper and continue to cook until heated through, about 4 minutes.

3 Reduce heat to low and add feta cheese. Stir to combine.

4 Cut a slit in the middle of each chicken breast to create a pocket. Spoon equal amounts of feta mixture into each breast. Secure with a toothpick.

5 Arrange chicken in a 9" × 13" baking dish. Bake for 35 minutes or until chicken is no longer pink and juices run clear. Serve warm.

Buffalo Chicken Zucchini Boats

BULK SHREDDED CHICKEN

It's helpful to make cooked meats in bulk and freeze in batches for recipes like this; a lot of recipes call for cooked chicken, for example. You can make a batch of shredded chicken in your slow cooker. Combine 1 teaspoon each salt, black pepper, garlic powder, and onion powder and sprinkle it over 3 pounds of boneless, skinless chicken breasts. Place chicken breasts in slow cooker, pour 1 cup chicken bone broth on top, and cook on low for 6 to 8 hours. Shred with two forks and store in the refrigerator for up to 1 week or freeze in batches.

Zucchini is a great vegetable source for your keto days, since one whole zucchini contains only 4 grams of net carbohydrates, and it has a mild flavor that pairs well with almost any topping. You can also replace the zucchini with yellow summer squash, which has a similar carbohydrate count.

2 large zucchini

2 tablespoons butter-flavored coconut oil

¼ cup minced peeled yellow onion

1 cup shredded cooked chicken

½ cup The New Primal buffalo sauce

¼ cup Tessemae's Organic Habanero Ranch dressing

1 large avocado, peeled, pitted, and diced

1 Preheat oven to 350°F.

2 Cut ends off zucchini and then slice each one in half lengthwise. Scoop out some of the flesh to create a "boat." Roughly chop the scooped zucchini and set aside.

3 Heat coconut oil in a medium skillet over medium heat. Add onion and cook for 2 minutes. Stir in chopped zucchini and cook for another 2 minutes or until slightly softened.

4 Add chicken to pan and stir to incorporate. Pour buffalo sauce on top of chicken mixture and stir until just combined.

5 Remove from heat. Arrange zucchini, cut side up, in a 9" × 13" baking dish. Scoop equal amounts of buffalo chicken into each zucchini boat and spread out evenly.

6 Bake for 20 minutes or until zucchini is tender. Remove from heat and drizzle ranch dressing over chicken. Top with avocado and serve.

Sesame Chicken

This Sesame Chicken pairs really well with a side of cauliflower rice and steamed broccoli. If you prefer, you can also cook everything together as a one-pot meal by adding the broccoli and cauliflower to the pan at the same time as the sauce and letting it cook until tender.

1 large egg

1 tablespoon arrowroot powder

1 pound boneless, skinless chicken thighs, cut into bite-sized pieces

3 tablespoons toasted sesame oil, divided

1 teaspoon sea salt

½ teaspoon ground black pepper

2 tablespoons coconut aminos

2 tablespoons golden monk fruit sweetener

1 tablespoon white vinegar

1 teaspoon minced garlic

2 tablespoons sesame seeds

SERVES 4	
Per Serving:	
Calories	252
Fat	17g
Protein	20g
Sodium	743mg
Fiber	1g
Carbohydrates	10g
Net Carbs	3g
Sugar	2g

1 Whisk together egg and arrowroot powder in a medium mixing bowl. Add chicken pieces and toss to coat completely.

2 Heat 2 tablespoons sesame oil in a medium skillet over medium-high heat. Add coated chicken and cook, flipping while cooking, until chicken is no longer pink, about 7 minutes.

3 Combine remaining sesame oil, salt, pepper, coconut aminos, monk fruit sweetener, vinegar, and garlic in a small bowl and whisk until smooth.

4 Pour sauce over chicken and stir. Reduce heat to low and continue cooking until thickened, about 3 minutes. Sprinkle sesame seeds on chicken and stir to combine.

5 Remove from heat and serve.

Baked Chicken Cordon Bleu

WHAT'S A PORK RIND?

Pork rind is just another term for pork skin. Commercial pork rinds are either fried or baked and then sold as a snack. Because they're so crispy and full of fat, they make a great substitute for bread crumbs on a keto diet. If you're using pork rinds, try to find some that are sourced from pigs that are pasture-raised and contain minimal ingredients.

The pork rinds give this chicken a crispy texture that's similar to the effect from panko bread crumbs. If you don't have any, or prefer not to use them, you can swap almond meal or paleo flour. The end result won't be as crispy, but it will still be delicious.

2 (2.5-ounce) bags baked pork rinds
½ teaspoon sea salt
¼ teaspoon ground black pepper
1 teaspoon Italian seasoning
¼ teaspoon granulated garlic
¼ teaspoon granulated onion
¼ teaspoon crushed red pepper
¼ cup grated Parmesan cheese
4 (4-ounce) boneless, skinless chicken breasts
8 slices no-sugar-added deli ham, thinly sliced
4 slices Swiss cheese
2 large eggs, lightly beaten

1 Preheat oven to 450°F. Line a baking sheet with parchment paper.

2 Combine pork rinds, salt, pepper, Italian seasoning, garlic, onion, red pepper, and Parmesan cheese in a food processor and pulse until crumbs form, about 1 minute. Transfer to a shallow dish.

3 Pound each chicken breast to ¼" thickness.

4 Layer two slices of deli ham and one slice of Swiss on each breast. Roll to close and secure in place with a toothpick.

5 Dip each rolled chicken breast in eggs and then roll in pork rind mixture, covering as much as possible. Transfer coated chicken breast to prepared baking sheet.

6 Bake for 25 minutes or until chicken is no longer pink and juices run clear. Cool slightly before serving.

Coconut Shrimp

If you don't have an air fryer, you can cook this shrimp on the stove by heating ¼ cup coconut oil over medium-high heat and then cooking for 3 minutes on each side or until shrimp turn pink.

2 large egg whites

¼ cup coconut flour

¼ teaspoon granulated garlic

¾ cup unsweetened shredded coconut

1 pound raw large shrimp, peeled and deveined

1 Preheat air fryer to 350°F.

2 Place egg whites in a medium bowl and beat on high speed with a handheld mixer until soft peaks form, about 4 minutes.

3 Combine coconut flour and garlic in a small bowl and place shredded coconut in a separate small bowl.

4 Dip each shrimp in coconut flour mixture, then egg whites, then shredded coconut.

5 Arrange shrimp in your air fryer and cook for 8 minutes or until shrimp turns pink.

6 Remove from air fryer and serve immediately.

SERVES 4	
Per Serving:	
Calories	240
Fat	12g
Protein	23g
Sodium	852mg
Fiber	5g
Carbohydrates	9g
Net Carbs	4g
Sugar	2g

SAVING YOUR YOLKS

Some recipes require only an egg white, but throwing away the yolk sends a lot of nutrients—like essential fatty acids and choline—right into the garbage. Instead of throwing away your yolks, you can use them to make homemade mayonnaise or hollandaise sauce for your Eggs Benedict and Baked Eggs Benedict recipes (see recipes in Chapter 2). You can also add a yolk to keto-friendly cookie recipes to give that sought-after chewiness or simply scramble them up with some vegetables!

Herb-Roasted Pork and Brussels Sprouts

Per Serving:

Calories	220
Fat	14g
Protein	18g
Sodium	737mg
Fiber	3g
Carbohydrates	6g
Net Carbs	3g
Sugar	1g

ALLOWING MEAT TO REST

You should always allow any meat to rest, or sit without cutting, for at least 10 minutes before you slice into it. If you slice it right after cooking, the juices haven't had a chance to settle back into the meat and will run out from the meat, all over your cutting board. If you let the meat rest, the juice stays in the meat, and you won't compromise any flavor.

Meat continues to cook for a few minutes after removing it from the oven because of the residual heat. Taking this pork roast out of the oven at 145°F will give you a medium-rare to medium roast. If you want your pork more well done, cook to 150°F–155°F.

3 tablespoons olive oil, divided

1 tablespoon Italian seasoning

½ teaspoon granulated garlic

1 teaspoon dried rosemary

2 teaspoons sea salt

1 teaspoon ground black pepper

1 (2-pound) pork tenderloin

2 tablespoons avocado oil

1 pound Brussels sprouts, trimmed and quartered

1 teaspoon lemon pepper

1 Preheat oven to 350°F. Line a baking sheet with parchment paper.

2 Combine 2 tablespoons olive oil, Italian seasoning, garlic, rosemary, salt, and pepper in a small bowl and mix well.

3 Rub mixture all over pork, covering as much as possible.

4 Heat avocado oil in a medium skillet over medium-high heat. Add pork to hot pan and brown on all sides, about 2 minutes per side.

5 Transfer pork to prepared baking sheet. Combine Brussels sprouts, remaining olive oil, and lemon pepper in a medium mixing bowl. Toss to coat.

6 Arrange Brussels sprouts around pork on baking sheet.

7 Cook for 30 minutes or until pork reaches an internal temperature of 145°F. Remove from oven and allow pork to rest for 10 minutes before slicing. Serve warm.

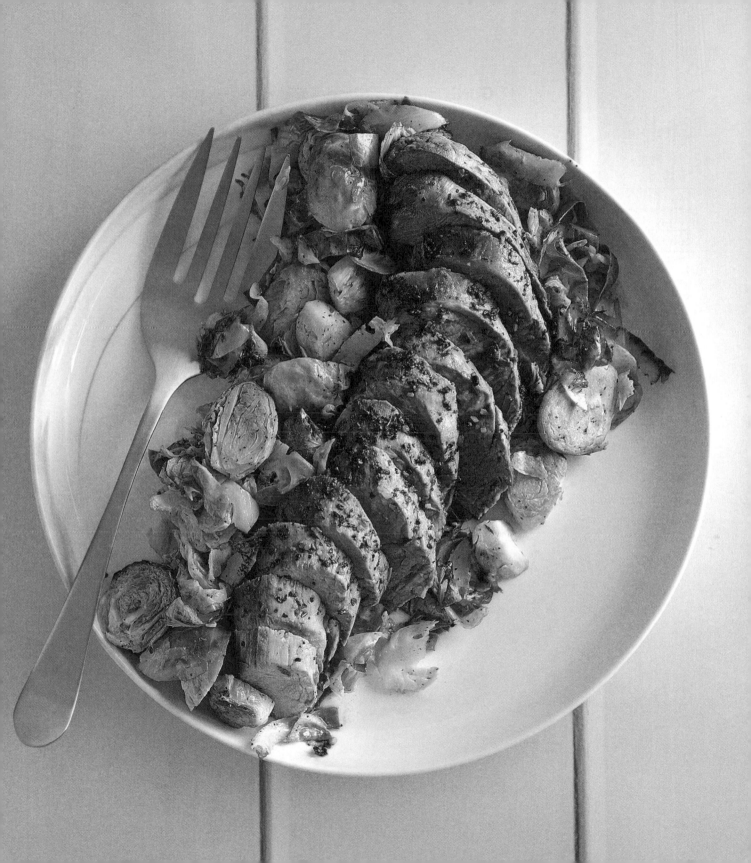

Garlic Butter Salmon and Asparagus

SERVES 4	
Per Serving:	
Calories	320
Fat	23g
Protein	21g
Sodium	570mg
Fiber	2g
Carbohydrates	4g
Net Carbs	2g
Sugar	2g

This Garlic Butter Salmon and Asparagus is a full meal on its own, but if you want to make it even heartier, combine it with Parmesan Herb Cauliflower (see recipe in Chapter 5). Asparagus is full of vitamins A, C, E, K, and B_6, plus it offers calcium, iron, and folate.

4 (4-ounce) salmon fillets

16 spears asparagus, trimmed

2 tablespoons minced garlic

1 tablespoon chopped fresh parsley

¼ cup lemon juice

¼ cup grass-fed butter, melted

1 teaspoon sea salt

½ teaspoon ground black pepper

1 Preheat oven to 400°F. Line a baking sheet with parchment paper.

2 Arrange salmon, skin side down, on prepared baking sheet. Surround salmon with trimmed asparagus.

3 Combine garlic and parsley in a small bowl and mash with a fork to mix. Spread mixture over salmon fillets.

4 In a separate small bowl, stir lemon juice and butter together. Pour mixture over salmon and asparagus. Sprinkle salt and pepper on top.

5 Bake for 10 minutes or until salmon flakes apart easily with a fork. Remove from oven and serve hot.

Creamy Chicken and Spinach Bake

This recipe calls for all the creamy ingredients—cream cheese, mayonnaise, and sour cream—that make a keto dish rich and full of that flavorful fat. If you don't have mayonnaise or sour cream, you can use 1 cup of one or the other.

8 ounces cream cheese, softened

½ cup keto-friendly mayonnaise

½ cup sour cream

1 teaspoon Dijon mustard

1 teaspoon fish sauce

2 teaspoons granulated garlic

2 teaspoons dried minced onion

1½ pounds cubed cooked chicken

1 (10-ounce) package frozen chopped spinach, thawed and drained

¾ cup grated Parmesan cheese

½ cup shredded mozzarella cheese

1 Preheat oven to 350°F.

2 Combine cream cheese, mayonnaise, sour cream, mustard, fish sauce, granulated garlic, and minced onion in a medium bowl and mix well.

3 Add chicken, spinach, and Parmesan cheese to cream cheese mixture and stir to combine.

4 Transfer mixture to a 9" × 13" baking dish. Sprinkle mozzarella cheese on top.

5 Bake for 35 minutes or until hot and bubbly. Remove from oven and allow to cool slightly before serving.

SERVES 6	
Per Serving:	
Calories	476
Fat	40g
Protein	24g
Sodium	938mg
Fiber	1g
Carbohydrates	7g
Net Carbs	6g
Sugar	3g

SHREDDING CHEESE

Many prepackaged cheeses contain cellulose, an insoluble fiber that comes from wood pulp and is impossible for humans to digest, and potato starch, which adds a small amount of carbohydrates. Manufacturers add them to prevent clumping, and although there haven't been any known negative side effects from either ingredient, shredding your own cheese may be a better option. If you prefer prepackaged cheese, read your ingredient lists and nutrition labels carefully.

Butter Steak with Garlic and Chives

SERVES 4

Per Serving:

Calories	287
Fat	20g
Protein	26g
Sodium	566mg
Fiber	0g
Carbohydrates	0g
Net Carbs	0g
Sugar	0g

DOES GRASS-FED MAKE A DIFFERENCE IN BUTTER?

Grass-fed isn't just a buzzword; cows that are raised on grass produce a butter that's much higher quality in taste and nutrition than cows raised on grain. Grass-fed butter is particularly rich in conjugated linoleic acid, or CLA—a fatty acid that helps fight cancer, prevents bone loss, and helps your body build muscle and burn fat. It's best if you're able to use grass-fed butter in any recipe that calls for it.

Adding the butter to the steak after cooking not only adds a load of healthy fats, but it also creates a soft texture that makes this steak melt in your mouth. If you don't have access to an outdoor grill, you can cook the steak in a skillet over medium heat instead.

1 tablespoon avocado oil

4 tablespoons grass-fed butter, softened

2 teaspoons minced garlic

2 teaspoons chopped fresh chives

1 teaspoon sea salt

½ teaspoon ground black pepper

1 pound sirloin steak

1 Preheat grill to high heat. Brush oil on grill grate.

2 Combine butter, garlic, and chives in a small bowl and stir to mix well.

3 Sprinkle salt and pepper on both sides of steak. Place steak on preheated grill and cook for 6 minutes on each side or until steak reaches desired level of doneness.

4 Remove steak from grill and brush with garlic butter mixture. Loosely cover with foil and allow to rest for 10 minutes.

5 Slice steak thinly and serve immediately.

Bacon-Wrapped Chicken Fingers

These Bacon-Wrapped Chicken Fingers are a delicious appetizer to bring to a party. If you want to make this recipe into a meal, serve with Twice-Baked Cauliflower, Parmesan Herb Cauliflower, or Garlic-Roasted Radishes (see recipes in Chapter 5).

1 pound chicken breast tenders (approximately 8 pieces)

½ teaspoon sea salt

½ teaspoon ground black pepper

½ teaspoon granulated garlic

4 slices Cheddar cheese, cut in half

8 slices no-sugar-added bacon

SERVES 4	
Per Serving:	
Calories	342
Fat	19g
Protein	39g
Sodium	1,236mg
Fiber	0g
Carbohydrates	1g
Net Carbs	1g
Sugar	0g

1 Preheat oven to 450°F. Line a baking sheet with parchment paper.

2 Arrange chicken tenders on baking sheet and sprinkle with salt, pepper, and garlic.

3 Place half of a cheese slice on top of each tender and wrap each piece in bacon. Secure with a toothpick.

4 Bake for 15 minutes or until chicken is no longer pink.

5 Remove from oven and serve warm.

Creamy Mushroom Chicken Thighs

SERVES 4	
Per Serving:	
Calories	457
Fat	39g
Protein	24g
Sodium	1,360mg
Fiber	1g
Carbohydrates	4g
Net Carbs	3g
Sugar	3g

Chicken thighs have more fat than chicken breasts, which gives this dish a richer flavor as well as a higher fat count. If you prefer chicken breasts, you can make the swap without losing much taste.

Chicken Thighs

1 teaspoon minced garlic

2 teaspoons dried rosemary

1 teaspoon sea salt

½ teaspoon ground black pepper

4 (4-ounce) boneless, skinless chicken thighs

2 tablespoons butter-flavored coconut oil

2 tablespoons lemon juice

Cream Sauce

1 tablespoon olive oil

1 cup sliced baby bella mushrooms

1 teaspoon minced garlic

2 teaspoons dried thyme

2 teaspoons chopped fresh parsley

½ teaspoon nutmeg

½ teaspoon Trader Joe's Mushroom & Company Multipurpose Umami Seasoning Blend

½ teaspoon sea salt

¼ teaspoon ground black pepper

¼ teaspoon crushed red pepper

1 cup heavy cream

½ cup shredded Parmesan cheese

1 **For Chicken Thighs:** Combine garlic, rosemary, sea salt, and black pepper in a small bowl. Mix well. Rub mixture on chicken thighs, covering as much as possible. Heat coconut oil in a medium skillet over medium-high heat. Add chicken to pan and cook for 7 minutes on each side or until chicken is cooked through. Remove from pan and sprinkle with lemon juice. Set aside.

2 **For Cream Sauce:** Reduce heat to medium and add olive oil and mushrooms to pan that was used to cook chicken thighs. Stir in garlic, thyme, parsley, nutmeg, umami seasoning blend, salt, black pepper, and red pepper. Cook for 1 minute. Stir in cream and bring to a simmer. Reduce heat to low and stir in Parmesan cheese. Add chicken to pan and spoon sauce over chicken. Simmer for 2 minutes. Remove from heat and serve.

Sweet and Salty Grilled Salmon

If you're in an area where it gets too cold to grill, you can cook this fish in the oven as well. Place fish on a parchment paper–lined baking sheet and bake at 350°F for about 12 minutes. Top with The Perfect Dill sauce, if desired.

1 teaspoon lemon pepper

2 teaspoons lemon juice

1 teaspoon granulated garlic

½ teaspoon sea salt

⅓ cup coconut aminos

⅓ cup golden monk fruit sweetener

⅓ cup chicken bone broth

4 (4-ounce) salmon fillets

¼ cup avocado oil

1 Combine lemon pepper, lemon juice, garlic, salt, coconut aminos, monk fruit sweetener, and broth in a resealable plastic bag. Massage to mix completely.

2 Add salmon to bag, making sure fish is coated. Refrigerate for 3 hours.

3 Preheat grill to medium heat.

4 Brush grill grate with oil.

5 Place fish flesh side down and cook for 7 minutes. Flip fish over, skin side down, for another 7 minutes or until salmon flakes easily with a fork.

6 Remove from grill and serve warm.

SERVES 4

Per Serving:

Calories	442
Fat	37g
Protein	21g
Sodium	826mg
Fiber	0g
Carbohydrates	22g
Net Carbs	6g
Sugar	5g

THE PERFECT DILL SAUCE

This dill sauce is perfect for grilled fish, baked fish, fish tacos, you name it; and it's so easy to make! Combine ½ cup full-fat Greek yogurt, ½ cup keto-friendly mayonnaise, 2 tablespoons lime juice, 1 minced jalapeño, ½ teaspoon dried oregano, ½ teaspoon ground cumin, ½ teaspoon dried dill weed, and ½ teaspoon cayenne pepper and whisk until smooth.

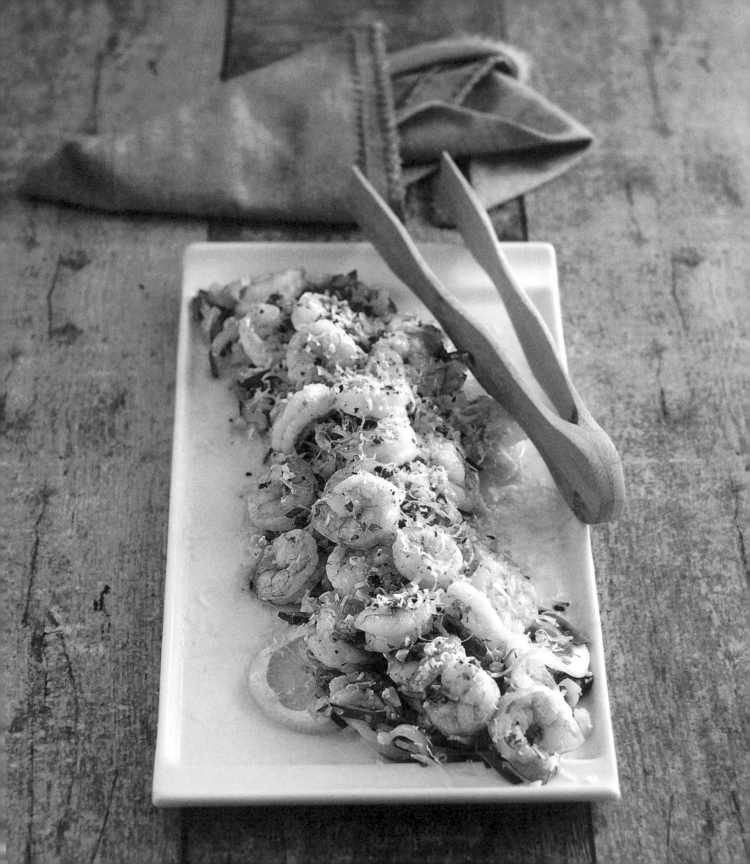

Garlic Butter Shrimp with Zoodles

This Garlic Butter Shrimp with Zoodles is the perfect weeknight dinner. It takes only one pan to make, and it's on the table in less than 30 minutes.

4 medium zucchini, spiralized

1½ teaspoons sea salt, divided

1 tablespoon olive oil

4 tablespoons grass-fed butter, divided

1 pound raw large shrimp, peeled and deveined

2 teaspoons minced garlic

½ teaspoon dried parsley

½ teaspoon dried basil

⅛ teaspoon crushed red pepper

1 tablespoon lemon juice

¼ cup chicken bone broth 2 teaspoons Frank's RedHot Original Cayenne Pepper Sauce

¼ teaspoon ground black pepper

¼ cup grated Parmesan cheese

SERVES 4	
Per Serving:	
Calories	308
Fat	19g
Protein	26g
Sodium	1,543mg
Fiber	2g
Carbohydrates	8g
Net Carbs	6g
Sugar	4g

1 Place spiralized zucchini in a strainer and sprinkle with 1 teaspoon salt. Toss to coat. Place strainer in the sink to let excess water drain out while preparing the rest of the recipe.

2 Heat olive oil and 2 tablespoons butter in a medium skillet over medium heat. Add shrimp and garlic and cook for 2 minutes. Add parsley, basil, and crushed red pepper, stir, and flip shrimp to uncooked side. Cook for 2 more minutes or until shrimp turn pink. Remove shrimp from pan and set aside.

3 Add lemon juice, broth, hot sauce, black pepper, and remaining salt and butter to pan and bring to a simmer, stirring constantly. Simmer for 3 minutes.

4 Add zucchini noodles to sauce and stir. Cook for 2 minutes. Stir in shrimp and remove from heat. Sprinkle Parmesan cheese on top. Serve immediately.

Buffalo Chicken Casserole

SERVES 4	
Per Serving:	
Calories	792
Fat	655g
Protein	36g
Sodium	1,896mg
Fiber	7g
Carbohydrates	19g
Net Carbs	12g
Sugar	6g

You can adjust the spiciness of this recipe by using either a mild, medium, or hot buffalo sauce. If you like things really spicy, you can add a pinch or two of cayenne pepper too.

2 tablespoons butter-flavored coconut oil

1 tablespoon minced garlic

1 medium yellow onion, peeled and chopped

1 cup chopped seeded orange bell pepper

2 cups broccoli slaw

2 cups riced cauliflower

½ teaspoon sea salt

¼ teaspoon ground black pepper

½ cup keto-friendly mayonnaise

½ cup sour cream, divided

½ cup The New Primal buffalo sauce

2 cups shredded cooked chicken

2 cups shredded sharp Cheddar cheese

1 large avocado, peeled, pitted, and sliced

1 Preheat oven to 375°F.

2 Heat coconut oil in a medium pan over medium heat. Add garlic and onions and cook for 2 minutes. Add bell peppers and broccoli slaw and cook until softened, about 4 minutes. Stir in cauliflower rice, salt, and black pepper and cook for another 4 minutes.

3 Transfer mixture to a 9" × 9" baking dish and spread out evenly.

4 Combine mayonnaise, ¼ cup sour cream, and buffalo sauce in a medium mixing bowl and whisk until smooth. Add chicken to mixture and toss to coat.

5 Spread chicken out on top of cauliflower mixture. Sprinkle cheese on top. Bake for 25 minutes or until bubbly and cheese starts to turn golden. Remove from heat and allow to cool slightly before serving.

6 Serve with remaining sour cream and avocado.

Roasted Beef Tenderloin

This Roasted Beef Tenderloin is so easy to make that it almost seems too good to be true—but it's not! Keep this recipe in mind for holiday get-togethers or when you really want to impress guests at a dinner party. As written, the beef tenderloin will be rare. If you prefer your meat more well done, cook it for a few more minutes.

¾ cup coconut aminos

½ cup grass-fed butter, melted

1 teaspoon granulated garlic

¼ teaspoon ground black pepper

1 (3-pound) beef tenderloin

1 Preheat oven to 350°F.

2 Combine coconut aminos, melted butter, garlic, and black pepper in a small bowl and whisk until smooth.

3 Place beef tenderloin in a 9" × 13" glass baking dish. Pour butter mixture over beef.

4 Bake for 10 minutes, flip tenderloin over, and bake for an additional 35 minutes or until internal temperature reaches 125°F.

5 Remove roast from oven and loosely place a piece of aluminum foil over tenderloin. Let sit for 15 minutes before slicing.

6 Serve warm.

SERVES 6	
Per Serving:	
Calories	622
Fat	44g
Protein	45g
Sodium	634mg
Fiber	0g
Carbohydrates	7g
Net Carbs	7g
Sugar	6g

Creamy Zoodles and Chicken

Per Serving:

Calories	380
Fat	29g
Protein	25g
Sodium	1,045mg
Fiber	2g
Carbohydrates	8g
Net Carbs	6g
Sugar	6g

The zucchini noodles in this recipe are cooked for a couple of minutes to soften them up and heat them through; but if you prefer your zucchini noodles a little crispier, place zoodles in a bowl, pour sauce on top, mix, then serve.

3 tablespoons grass-fed butter, divided

1 pound boneless, skinless chicken thighs, cubed

1 teaspoon garlic salt

1 teaspoon minced garlic

4 ounces cream cheese

3 tablespoons heavy cream

¼ cup grated Parmesan cheese

4 medium zucchini, spiralized

½ teaspoon sea salt

½ teaspoon ground black pepper

1 Heat 2 tablespoons butter in a medium skillet over medium heat. Add chicken pieces and sprinkle with garlic salt. Stir to mix.

2 Cook until chicken is no longer pink, about 7 minutes. Remove chicken from pan and set aside.

3 Reduce heat to low and add remaining butter to pan. Stir in garlic and cook for 1 minute. Add cream cheese and cream and stir until melted.

4 Once melted, add Parmesan cheese and stir until smooth. Stir in zucchini, salt, and pepper and cook for 2 minutes.

5 Remove from heat and serve.

Cajun Shrimp "Pasta"

This recipe calls for cooked spaghetti squash, but you can serve the shrimp and cream sauce over any other keto-friendly pasta substitute. Zucchini noodles work well too!

2 tablespoons grass-fed butter

½ cup minced seeded green bell pepper

1½ cups heavy cream

2 tablespoons chopped fresh basil

1 tablespoon dried parsley

1½ teaspoons sea salt

2 teaspoons ground black pepper

1 teaspoon crushed red pepper

⅛ teaspoon cayenne pepper

⅓ cup chopped green onion

1½ pounds raw large shrimp, peeled and deveined

½ cup grated Parmesan cheese

½ cup shredded mozzarella cheese

3 cups cooked spaghetti squash

SERVES 6	
Per Serving:	
Calories	442
Fat	33g
Protein	29g
Sodium	1,599mg
Fiber	2g
Carbohydrates	10g
Net Carbs	8g
Sugar	4g

1 Heat butter in a large skillet over medium heat. Add bell peppers and cook until slightly softened, about 3 minutes.

2 Add cream to skillet and bring to a light boil. Reduce heat to low and add basil, parsley, salt, black pepper, red pepper, cayenne pepper, and green onions. Simmer for 30 minutes.

3 Add shrimp and simmer until shrimp turn pink, about 7 minutes. Stir in Parmesan cheese and mozzarella cheese.

4 Add spaghetti squash and toss to coat. Cook until heated through, about 3 minutes.

5 Remove from heat and serve.

Parmesan-Crusted Cod

SERVES 4

Per Serving:

Calories	214
Fat	13g
Protein	23g
Sodium	358mg
Fiber	0g
Carbohydrates	1g
Net Carbs	1g
Sugar	0g

This Parmesan crust works well with any mild white fish, so you can try it with haddock or sea bass as well. Serve it with some roasted vegetables tossed in grass-fed butter for a complete keto meal.

¼ **cup grated Parmesan cheese**

2 **tablespoons grass-fed butter, softened**

1½ **tablespoons keto-friendly mayonnaise**

1 **tablespoon lemon juice**

¼ **teaspoon dried basil**

¼ **teaspoon sea salt**

¼ **teaspoon ground black pepper**

¼ **teaspoon granulated onion**

¼ **teaspoon granulated garlic**

¼ **teaspoon paprika**

⅛ **teaspoon celery seed**

4 **(4-ounce) cod fillets**

1 Preheat oven broiler to high. Line a baking sheet with parchment paper.

2 Combine Parmesan cheese, butter, mayonnaise, lemon juice, basil, salt, pepper, onion, garlic, paprika, and celery seed in a small bowl and mix well.

3 Arrange cod fillets on prepared baking sheet and broil for 2 minutes. Flip fish over, spread Parmesan mixture onto fillets, and broil for another 3 minutes or until Parmesan crust starts to brown and fish flakes apart easily with a fork.

4 Serve immediately.

Blackened Cajun Chicken

This Blackened Cajun Chicken has some serious kick. If you prefer it a little less spicy, reduce the amount of cayenne pepper and/or omit the red pepper flakes.

1½ teaspoons paprika

¾ teaspoon ground cumin

¼ teaspoon dried thyme

½ teaspoon granulated onion

¼ teaspoon granulated garlic

¼ teaspoon sea salt

¼ teaspoon ground black pepper

½ teaspoon cayenne pepper

¼ teaspoon crushed red pepper

2 tablespoons avocado oil

4 (4-ounce) boneless, skinless chicken breasts

1 Preheat oven to 350°F.

2 Combine all spices in a large resealable plastic bag.

3 Brush oil on chicken breasts and add chicken to bag. Shake to coat chicken.

4 Heat a medium cast iron skillet over high heat for 5 minutes.

5 Add chicken to hot pan and cook for 1 minute. Turn, then cook for another minute.

6 Transfer skillet to preheated oven and bake for 5 minutes or until chicken is no longer pink and juices run clear. Serve warm.

SERVES 4

Per Serving:

Calories	197
Fat	10g
Protein	24g
Sodium	513mg
Fiber	1g
Carbohydrates	1g
Net Carbs	0g
Sugar	0g

CLEANING CAST IRON

Did you know there's a "right" way to clean your cast iron cookware? Using the dishwasher or regular dish soap can strip the pan's seasoning, compromising the taste of any food you cook on it. To properly clean cast iron, mix kosher salt and water in the pan and use a rag to scrub off any stuck-on bits with the paste. Once any food particles are removed, rinse and then wipe salt away with a paper towel. For stubborn messes, you can boil some water in the pan on the stove before scrubbing.

Chicken Piccata

This classic dish can easily be converted for a keto diet. You can serve this Chicken Piccata alongside your favorite vegetable or on top of any keto-friendly pasta substitute, like spaghetti squash or zoodles. When preparing the chicken, you'll coat it with flour before and after dipping it into the egg mixture. This thickens the breading and makes it nice and crispy.

SERVES 4

Per Serving:

Calories	256
Fat	17g
Protein	21g
Sodium	489mg
Fiber	1g
Carbohydrates	5g
Net Carbs	4g
Sugar	1g

COUNTING THE CAPERS

Capers are immature flower buds that come from the *Capparis spinosa*, also called the *caper bush*. Just like olives, they're native to the Mediterranean region. Capers add a fresh saltiness with minimal carbohydrates to any dish. Two tablespoons, which is really all you need, contain only 0.8 grams of carbohydrates, 0.6 of which come from fiber.

1 large egg

3 tablespoons lemon juice, divided

¼ cup paleo flour

½ teaspoon lemon zest

¼ teaspoon granulated garlic

⅛ teaspoon paprika

½ teaspoon sea salt

4 (4-ounce) boneless, skinless chicken thighs

¼ cup grass-fed butter

½ cup chicken bone broth

2 tablespoons capers

1 Whisk together egg and 1 tablespoon lemon juice in a small mixing bowl. In a shallow bowl, combine paleo flour, lemon zest, garlic, paprika, and salt.

2 Dip each chicken thigh in flour mixture, coating completely, then dip coated chicken in egg mixture and then flour mixture again.

3 Heat butter in a medium skillet over medium heat. Add chicken and cook for 3 minutes on each side or until browned (chicken doesn't have to be completely cooked).

4 Add broth and remaining lemon juice to the skillet. Stir in capers and reduce heat to low. Simmer for 20 minutes or until chicken is cooked through, turning chicken once while cooking.

5 Remove from heat and serve.

Marinated Shrimp Skillet

When planning your dinner, keep in mind that shrimp requires at least 2 hours of marinating. Giving the shrimp the proper time to marinate will really boost the flavor of the finished dish.

½ cup olive oil

½ cup grass-fed butter, melted

¼ cup chopped fresh parsley

2 tablespoons lemon juice

2 tablespoons Frank's RedHot Original Cayenne Pepper Sauce

2 teaspoons minced garlic

1 tablespoon no-sugar-added ketchup

1 teaspoon dried oregano

1 teaspoon sea salt

1 teaspoon ground black pepper

¼ teaspoon crushed red pepper

1½ pounds raw large shrimp, peeled and deveined

1 Preheat oven to 425°F.

2 Combine all ingredients except shrimp in a small bowl and whisk until smooth. Place mixture and shrimp in a resealable plastic bag. Seal and refrigerate for 2 hours.

3 After 2 hours, transfer shrimp and marinade into a medium oven-safe skillet. Bake for 30 minutes, stirring mixture once while cooking.

4 Remove from oven and serve.

SERVES 6	
Per Serving:	
Calories	412
Fat	35g
Protein	21g
Sodium	1,387mg
Fiber	0g
Carbohydrates	3g
Net Carbs	3g
Sugar	0g

Cauliflower Rice Pizza Bake

SERVES 4

Per Serving:

Calories	486
Fat	30g
Protein	34g
Sodium	1,793mg
Fiber	6g
Carbohydrates	17g
Net Carbs	11g
Sugar	8g

If you don't have any cauliflower rice on hand, you can also make this Cauliflower Rice Pizza Bake with small florets of cauliflower in its place. It's delicious with broccoli as well, but the broccoli adds a stronger flavor than the cauliflower does.

2 tablespoons olive oil

2 teaspoons minced garlic

1 medium yellow onion, peeled and diced

1 (12-ounce) bag frozen riced cauliflower

¼ cup finely minced seeded green bell pepper

1 pound 85/15 ground beef

1½ tablespoons Italian seasoning

1 teaspoon granulated garlic

1½ teaspoons sea salt

1 teaspoon ground black pepper

1½ cups no-sugar-added pizza sauce

½ cup shredded mozzarella cheese

½ cup shredded sharp Cheddar cheese

¼ cup grated Parmesan cheese

¼ teaspoon dried basil

1 Preheat oven to 375°F.

2 Heat olive oil in a medium skillet over medium-high heat. Add minced garlic and onion and cook for 2 minutes. Add riced cauliflower and bell peppers and cook for an additional 5 minutes.

3 Add ground beef and cook for 2 minutes. Stir in Italian seasoning, granulated garlic, salt, and black pepper and continue cooking until beef is no longer pink, about 5 minutes.

4 Transfer mixture to an 8" × 8" baking dish.

5 Pour pizza sauce on top and spread out evenly. Sprinkle mozzarella and Cheddar cheeses over pizza sauce, then top with Parmesan cheese and basil.

6 Bake for 25 minutes or until hot and bubbly and cheese is melted. Allow to cool slightly before serving.

CHAPTER 5

Keto Side Dishes

Fresh Broccoli Slaw

SERVES 6

Per Serving:

Calories	108
Fat	11g
Protein	1g
Sodium	367mg
Fiber	1g
Carbohydrates	6g
Net Carbs	2g
Sugar	1g

DON'T THROW AWAY THOSE BROCCOLI STEMS!

Many grocery stores carry bagged broccoli slaw in the refrigerated section of the produce department. If you can't find bagged broccoli slaw, or you need a great way to repurpose your broccoli stems so they don't go to waste, you can make your own slaw from stems. Remove broccoli stems from broccoli bunches and use a cheese grater to shred into matchsticks. A 12-ounce bag of broccoli slaw is equivalent to approximately 5 cups of shredded broccoli stems.

If you're making this Fresh Broccoli Slaw for one of your higher-carb days, you can throw in some raisins to add a complementary sweetness to the dish.

⅓ **cup keto-friendly mayonnaise**

1 **tablespoon apple cider vinegar**

1 **tablespoon Dijon mustard**

1½ **tablespoons granulated erythritol**

½ **teaspoon sea salt**

¼ **teaspoon ground black pepper**

1 **(12-ounce) bag broccoli slaw**

1 Whisk mayonnaise, apple cider vinegar, mustard, erythritol, salt, and black pepper together in a medium bowl.

2 Add broccoli slaw and toss to coat.

3 Refrigerate for 1 hour before serving.

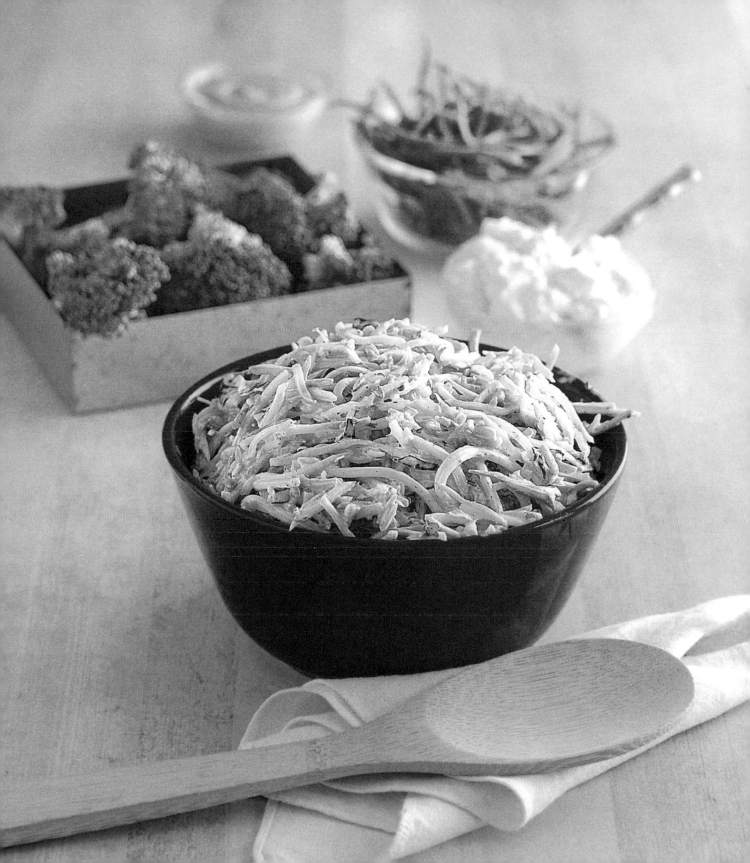

Greek Cauliflower Rice

SERVES 4	
Per Serving:	
Calories	98
Fat	7g
Protein	3g
Sodium	279mg
Fiber	3g
Carbohydrates	7g
Net Carbs	4g
Sugar	4g

This Greek Cauliflower Rice pairs well with Greek Lemon Chicken (see recipe in Chapter 8).

2 tablespoons olive oil

1 teaspoon minced garlic

1 small red onion, peeled and minced

1 medium green bell pepper, seeded and minced

1 (12-ounce) bag frozen riced cauliflower

1 teaspoon Greek seasoning

½ teaspoon sea salt

¼ teaspoon ground black pepper

1 Heat oil in a medium skillet over medium heat. Add garlic and onion and sauté 3 minutes. Add bell pepper and cook 3 more minutes.

2 Add cauliflower and cook until it starts to soften, about 4 minutes. Stir in Greek seasoning, salt, and black pepper and cook another 2 minutes or until slightly golden. Serve hot.

Parmesan Asparagus

SERVES 6	
Per Serving:	
Calories	127
Fat	15g
Protein	6g
Sodium	496mg
Fiber	2g
Carbohydrates	4g
Net Carbs	2g
Sugar	2g

You can whip up this Parmesan Asparagus with a handful of ingredients that you probably already have on hand. It's an easy side dish that tastes great alongside any protein dish.

¼ cup grass-fed butter

2 tablespoons olive oil

1¼ pounds asparagus, trimmed

½ cup grated Parmesan cheese

1 teaspoon sea salt

½ teaspoon ground black pepper

¼ teaspoon crushed red pepper

1 Heat a large skillet over medium heat. Add butter and olive oil. Once butter is melted and mixture is hot, add asparagus and cook until tender but still slightly crisp, about 10 minutes.

2 Drain excess oil. Add remaining ingredients and toss to coat. Serve hot.

Chicken Parmesan Dip

This Chicken Parmesan Dip is so good that you're going to want to eat it right from the dish with a spoon. Although that's certainly keto-friendly, you could also try scooping it up with some raw zucchini slices, which have a crisp texture and mild taste.

½ cup coarse almond meal

1 teaspoon Italian seasoning

2 tablespoons grated Parmesan cheese

1 (12.5-ounce) can white chunk chicken breast

8 ounces cream cheese, softened

1 cup no-sugar-added marinara sauce, divided

1 cup shredded mozzarella cheese

SERVES 12	
Per Serving:	
Calories	218
Fat	17g
Protein	12g
Sodium	371mg
Fiber	1g
Carbohydrates	5g
Net Carbs	4g
Sugar	2g

1 Preheat oven to 350°F.

2 Combine almond meal, Italian seasoning, and Parmesan cheese in a medium bowl. Add chicken and toss to coat.

3 Spread cream cheese in the bottom of an 8" × 8" baking dish. Spread ½ cup marinara sauce on cream cheese and top with chicken mixture.

4 Pour remaining sauce evenly over chicken and sprinkle mozzarella cheese on top.

5 Bake for 30 minutes or until hot and bubbly. Remove from oven and allow to cool slightly before serving.

Spicy Parmesan Broccoli Rabe

IT ISN'T BROCCOLI!

Although the name might understandably have you fooled, broccoli rabe isn't related to broccoli. The leafy, bitter green is actually more closely related to the turnip. Broccoli rabe is one of the most keto-friendly vegetables, clocking in at only 1.1 grams of carbohydrates per 1-cup serving. What's more, almost 100 percent of the carbohydrates in broccoli rabe come from fiber, so the green vegetable supplies a boatload of nutrients without affecting your blood sugar.

Boiling broccoli rabe in water before sautéing it in some oil helps cut the bitterness down a little bit. Don't skip this step! The end result is worth the few minutes of extra time.

½ teaspoon sea salt

1 pound broccoli rabe, trimmed

4 tablespoons grass-fed butter

2 teaspoons minced garlic

½ teaspoon crushed red pepper

1 tablespoon grated Parmesan cheese

1 Add salt to a large pot of water. Bring water to a boil over medium-high heat.

2 Add broccoli rabe to boiling water and cook until tender but still slightly crispy, about 4 minutes. Drain.

3 While broccoli rabe is cooking, heat butter in a medium skillet over medium heat. Add garlic and cook for 1 minute.

4 Add broccoli rabe to skillet and cook for 10 minutes or until softened.

5 Combine crushed red pepper and Parmesan cheese in a small bowl and sprinkle over broccoli rabe. Toss to coat.

6 Remove from heat and serve.

Shredded Brussels Sprouts with Bacon

Think you don't like Brussels sprouts? This recipe will change your mind! If you have extra time, you can soak the Brussels sprouts for an hour in salt water before shredding them to cut some of their characteristic bitterness.

6 slices no-sugar-added bacon

3 tablespoons grass-fed butter

½ teaspoon minced garlic

¼ cup pine nuts

2 (10-ounce) bags shaved Brussels sprouts

2 green onions, minced

½ teaspoon seasoning salt

¼ teaspoon ground black pepper

1 tablespoon grated Parmesan cheese

1 Heat a large skillet over medium-high heat. Add bacon and cook until crispy, about 7 minutes, flipping once. Transfer bacon to a paper towel–lined plate.

2 Reserve 2 tablespoons of bacon grease and dispose of the rest safely. Add butter to pan and allow to melt. Add garlic and cook for 30 seconds before adding pine nuts. Cook until pine nuts start to brown, about 3 minutes.

3 Add Brussels sprouts, green onions, salt, and pepper to the pan and cook until Brussels sprouts are tender but still slightly crispy, about 8 minutes.

4 While Brussels sprouts are cooking, roughly chop bacon.

5 When Brussels sprouts are tender, stir in bacon and Parmesan cheese. Serve hot.

SERVES 6	
Per Serving:	
Calories	233
Fat	19g
Protein	8g
Sodium	393mg
Fiber	4g
Carbohydrates	10g
Net Carbs	6g
Sugar	2g

BENEFITS OF BRUSSELS SPROUTS

Brussels sprouts are classified as cruciferous vegetables, along with kale, cauliflower, broccoli, and mustard greens. A ½ cup of the mini cabbages contains only 4 net carbohydrates, but more than the recommended daily intake (RDI) for vitamin K and more than 75 percent the RDI for vitamin C. Brussels sprouts are especially high in a compound called *kaempferol*, an antioxidant that may help reduce the growth of cancer cells, reduce inflammation, and boost heart health.

Lemon Butter Zucchini

Zucchini isn't just one of the go-to vegetables on the keto diet because it's low in carbs; it's also because of its mild flavor. Because zucchini doesn't have an overpowering taste, it lends well to lots of different flavor combinations, like this simple marriage of lemon and dill.

SERVES 6	
Per Serving:	
Calories	96
Fat	8g
Protein	2g
Sodium	14mg
Fiber	1g
Carbohydrates	5g
Net Carbs	4g
Sugar	4g

3 large zucchini, cut into ½″ rounds

¼ cup grass-fed butter, melted

1½ tablespoons lemon pepper

1 teaspoon dried dill

1 Preheat oven to 400°F. Line a baking sheet with parchment paper.

2 Arrange zucchini slices on baking sheet and brush with melted butter. Sprinkle lemon pepper and dill on top.

3 Bake for 20 minutes or until tender. Serve hot.

Curried Cauliflower

The curry powder gives this Curried Cauliflower a nice little kick that pairs well with Blackened Cajun Chicken and Baked Mustard Salmon (see recipes in Chapter 4). This hands-off recipe is easy to make while you prepare one of the main dishes.

SERVES 6	
Per Serving:	
Calories	157
Fat	16g
Protein	2g
Sodium	359mg
Fiber	2g
Carbohydrates	5g
Net Carbs	3g
Sugar	1g

½ cup keto-friendly mayonnaise

2 tablespoons curry powder

½ teaspoon sea salt

1 large head cauliflower, cut into florets

1 Preheat oven to 375°F. Line a baking sheet with parchment paper.

2 Whisk together mayonnaise, curry powder, and salt in a medium mixing bowl. Add cauliflower florets and toss to coat.

3 Arrange cauliflower on prepared baking sheet and bake for 30 minutes or until cauliflower is tender. Serve hot.

Sautéed Swiss Chard

Swiss chard may not be something you reach for often, but you should make it a regular part of your keto lifestyle. The more greens you include, the greater variety of micronutrients you'll get.

2 bunches Swiss chard

½ cup water

8 slices no-sugar-added bacon, chopped

¼ cup grass-fed butter

2 teaspoons minced garlic

⅓ cup fresh lemon juice

1 teaspoon sea salt

½ teaspoon ground black pepper

1 Remove leaves from Swiss chard stems. Roughly chop leaves and dice stems.

2 Add water and diced stems to a small saucepan. Cook over low heat until stems are tender, about 6 minutes. Drain water and set aside.

3 Cook bacon in a medium skillet over medium-high heat until it starts to crisp, about 5 minutes. Add butter to skillet. When butter is melted, add garlic and cook for 30 seconds. Pour lemon juice into the pan and use a wooden spoon to scrape any browned bits from the bottom of the pan.

4 Add Swish chard leaves and cook for 1 minute or until leaves start to wilt. Cover and cook for an additional 4 minutes. Add cooked stems, salt, and pepper, then stir and cook for an additional minute. Serve hot.

SERVES 6

Per Serving:

Calories	150
Fat	13g
Protein	5g
Sodium	742mg
Fiber	1g
Carbohydrates	4g
Net Carbs	3g
Sugar	1g

THE LOWDOWN ON SWISS CHARD

Swiss chard is high in an antioxidant called *alpha-lipoic acid*. Research shows that alpha-lipoic acid can reduce insulin resistance—a complication of eating too many of the wrong types of carbs that can eventually lead to diabetes. People with the highest intake of leafy green vegetables rich in alpha-lipoic acid have a 13 percent lower risk of developing diabetes than those with lower intakes.

Buffalo Cauliflower

SERVES 6

Per Serving:

Calories	95
Fat	8g
Protein	4g
Sodium	770mg
Fiber	2g
Carbohydrates	5g
Net Carbs	3g
Sugar	2g

Buffalo flavor is a crowd-pleaser, so this recipe is a good way to get people who don't love cauliflower interested in eating it. If you want to add a few more grams of fat to this side dish, drizzle some keto-friendly ranch dressing, like Tessemae's Organic Creamy Ranch Dressing, on top, along with some chopped avocados.

½ cup Frank's RedHot Original Cayenne Pepper Sauce

3 tablespoons grass-fed butter

1 large head cauliflower, cut into florets

½ teaspoon granulated garlic

½ teaspoon granulated onion

¼ cup grated Parmesan cheese

1 Preheat oven to 375°F. Line a baking sheet with parchment paper.

2 Combine hot sauce and butter in a small saucepan and stir over low heat until melted and smooth.

3 Transfer sauce to a medium bowl and add cauliflower florets. Toss to coat. Sprinkle garlic and onion on top of cauliflower and toss to coat again.

4 Arrange cauliflower on baking sheet and bake for 30 minutes. Sprinkle Parmesan cheese on top of cauliflower and bake for an additional 5 minutes.

5 Remove from oven and serve hot.

Green Beans with Bacon

Use fresh green beans for this recipe instead of frozen beans. The fresh beans will give you a nice crispy outcome, while the frozen beans have a mushier texture that becomes overdone quickly.

6 slices no-sugar-added bacon, chopped

¼ cup minced peeled yellow onion

1 teaspoon minced garlic

1 pound fresh green beans, trimmed

1 cup chicken bone broth

¼ teaspoon sea salt

¼ teaspoon ground black pepper

1 Heat a medium skillet over medium-high heat. Add bacon and cook until fat begins to render, about 3 minutes. Add onion and garlic and cook for 1 minute. Stir in beans and broth.

2 Cook for 8 minutes or until beans are tender and broth has evaporated. Add salt and pepper and stir to combine. Serve hot.

SERVES 6

Per Serving:

Calories	75
Fat	4g
Protein	5g
Sodium	314mg
Fiber	3g
Carbohydrates	5g
Net Carbs	2g
Sugar	2g

GREEN BEANS: THE VEGETABLE THAT ISN'T

Although often classified as a vegetable, green beans actually belong to the legume family (along with beans and lentils). Unlike other legumes, however, green beans are low in carbohydrates. One cup of green beans contains about 7 grams of carbohydrates, 3.4 grams of which come from fiber. Green beans also contain carotenoids, which help improve brain function and protect brain health during aging.

Zucchini Pizza Bites

This recipe is an excellent way to use up all that extra zucchini growing in your garden. (The larger the zucchini, the better!) These Zucchini Pizza bites will go quickly!

2 large zucchini, cut into rounds

¼ cup grass-fed butter, melted

1 teaspoon minced garlic

⅔ cup no-sugar-added pizza sauce

⅔ cup shredded mozzarella cheese

2 tablespoons grated Parmesan cheese

1 Preheat oven to 350°F. Line a baking sheet with parchment paper.

2 Arrange zucchini slices in a single layer on prepared baking sheet.

3 Combine melted butter and garlic in a small bowl. Brush butter mixture on each zucchini round. Flip rounds over and brush butter mixture on other side.

4 Scoop equal amounts of pizza sauce onto each round. Add mozzarella cheese on top of pizza sauce and sprinkle with Parmesan cheese.

5 Bake for 25 minutes or until zucchini is tender and cheese is hot and bubbly.

6 Remove from oven and serve immediately.

Cheesy Artichoke Casserole

Quartered artichoke hearts contain 6 grams of carbohydrates per ½ cup. Since 2.7 of those grams come from fiber, the net carbohydrate count is only 3.3 grams per serving, which classifies them as a low-carb vegetable.

2 (10-ounce) cans quartered artichoke hearts, drained

¾ cup grated Parmesan cheese

2 teaspoons granulated garlic

½ cup keto-friendly mayonnaise

1 tablespoon dried parsley

1 tablespoon dried minced onion

½ teaspoon paprika

1 Preheat oven to 350°F.

2 Combine artichoke hearts, Parmesan cheese, garlic, mayonnaise, parsley, and onion in a medium mixing bowl and stir until combined.

3 Transfer mixture to an 8" × 8" baking dish and sprinkle paprika on top.

4 Bake for 25 minutes or until bubbly. Serve hot.

SERVES 6	
Per Serving:	
Calories	252
Fat	21g
Protein	10g
Sodium	967mg
Fiber	2g
Carbohydrates	12g
Net Carbs	10g
Sugar	0g

FEEDING YOUR GOOD BACTERIA

An artichoke is unique in the type of fiber it contains. A percentage of the fiber content in an artichoke comes from inulin, which acts as a prebiotic—a compound that feeds good gut bacteria and contributes to a healthy gut. Regularly eating artichokes can keep your gut's ecosystem balanced.

Sausage and Green Beans

SERVES 8

Per Serving:

Calories	255
Fat	19g
Protein	12g
Sodium	443mg
Fiber	4g
Carbohydrates	9g
Net Carbs	5g
Sugar	3g

This recipe serves eight as a side dish, but if you want to make it a meal, you can increase the portion size and add some healthy fats, like a couple tablespoons of a keto-friendly dressing.

1 tablespoon olive oil

1 small shallot, peeled and minced

2 teaspoons minced garlic

1 pound no-sugar-added spicy pork sausage

1 cup beef bone broth

2 pounds fresh green beans, trimmed

1 teaspoon seasoning salt

1 Heat olive oil in a large saucepan over medium heat. Add shallot and garlic and cook for 1 minute. Add sausage and cook until no longer pink, about 7 minutes.

2 Pour in beef broth and stir, scraping the bottom of the saucepan with a wooden spoon to release any browned bits.

3 Add green beans and reduce heat to medium-low. Cover and simmer for 25 minutes or until green beans are tender.

4 Remove from heat and sprinkle with seasoning salt, tossing to coat. Serve hot.

Simmered Collard Greens

Collard greens, an excellent source of B vitamins, vitamin E, iron, and copper, are a Southern favorite that are low in carbohydrates and high in vitamins, minerals, and antioxidants. Work them into your keto lifestyle with other leafy greens as much as you can to get the most nutrition possible.

4 cups chicken bone broth

2 cups water

1 pound ham hocks

4 pounds collard greens, trimmed and roughly chopped

1 teaspoon crushed red pepper

¼ cup olive oil

½ teaspoon sea salt

¼ teaspoon ground black pepper

1 teaspoon red wine vinegar

1   Combine broth, water, and ham hocks in a large pot and bring to a boil over high heat. Lower heat to low and simmer for 30 minutes.

2   Add collard greens and red pepper to the pot, stir, and cover. Simmer for 2 hours, stirring occasionally.

3   Stir in olive oil and simmer, covered, for another 30 minutes.

4   Remove from heat and sprinkle salt, pepper, and red wine vinegar on top. Serve hot.

SERVES 6	
Per Serving:	
Calories	224
Fat	12g
Protein	17g
Sodium	459mg
Fiber	12g
Carbohydrates	17g
Net Carbs	5g
Sugar	1g

A HAM WHAT?

A ham hock, also called a *pork knuckle*, is the lower leg of a pig. It adds a smoky, salty flavor to what you're cooking it in. Typically, you find it cured or smoked in the meat section next to the pork products. If you can't find a ham hock, you can replace it with 4 ounces of chopped salted pork, 4 ounces of chopped smoked bacon, or 4 ounces of chopped smoked ham.

Bacon and Feta Asparagus

SERVES 6	
Per Serving:	
Calories	146
Fat	12g
Protein	7g
Sodium	401mg
Fiber	2g
Carbohydrates	4g
Net Carbs	2g
Sugar	1g

This unique take on asparagus combines several interesting flavor profiles. If you're sensitive to cow's milk, you can swap the feta cheese in this recipe for crumbled goat cheese, which gives it a creamy, salty flavor without any of the bothersome proteins.

3 tablespoons grass-fed butter, melted

¼ teaspoon sea salt

½ teaspoon ground black pepper

1 large bunch asparagus, trimmed

6 slices no-sugar-added bacon, cooked and chopped

¾ cup crumbled feta cheese

1 Preheat oven to 450°F. Line a baking sheet with parchment paper.

2 Whisk together butter, salt, and pepper in a large mixing bowl. Add asparagus and toss to coat.

3 Arrange asparagus in a single layer on prepared baking sheet. Bake until tender, about 10 minutes.

4 Sprinkle cooked bacon and feta on top and stir to coat. Serve immediately.

Jalapeño Popper Mashed Cauliflower

This Jalapeño Popper Mashed Cauliflower gives you all the spicy, creamy taste of jalapeño poppers but without the hassle of stuffing, filling, and wrapping them. You can stir in some crispy bacon after puréeing to kick the flavor up a notch.

1 large head cauliflower, cut into florets

½ cup water

¼ cup grass-fed butter

1 medium jalapeño, seeded and minced

3 green onions, finely chopped

1 teaspoon minced garlic

4 ounces cream cheese, softened

¼ cup sour cream

½ teaspoon sea salt

¼ teaspoon ground black pepper

1 Combine cauliflower and water in a large pot over medium heat. Allow cauliflower to steam until soft, about 8 minutes. Drain water and transfer cauliflower to a food processor.

2 Heat butter in a small skillet over medium heat. Add jalapeños, green onions, and garlic and cook until softened, about 3 minutes.

3 Add butter mixture to food processor along with cream cheese, sour cream, salt, and black pepper. Pulse until smooth, about 2 minutes.

4 Serve immediately.

SERVES 6

Per Serving:

Calories	178
Fat	16g
Protein	3g
Sodium	259mg
Fiber	2g
Carbohydrates	6g
Net Carbs	4g
Sugar	3g

A CANCER-FIGHTING CHILI PEPPER?

The capsaicin in peppers like jalapeños doesn't just help boost metabolism. A study from the Luohe Medical College in China found that capsaicin may even help stop tumor growth by affecting protein function. Other research shows that capsaicin also targets genes that suppress tumors.

White Mushroom Bake

SERVES 6

Per Serving:

Calories	227
Fat	17g
Protein	11g
Sodium	237mg
Fiber	2g
Carbohydrates	10g
Net Carbs	8g
Sugar	5g

Mushrooms are an excellent keto-friendly vegetable choice, with 1 cup containing only 2.3 grams of carbohydrates. Combine this White Mushroom Bake with a green vegetable and a protein to make a complete low-carb-day meal.

2 tablespoons grass-fed butter

1 medium yellow onion, peeled and diced

7 cups quartered white button mushrooms

1 cup sour cream

½ teaspoon sea salt

¼ teaspoon ground black pepper

1 cup shredded Swiss cheese

1 Preheat oven to 425°F.

2 Heat butter in a large skillet over medium heat. Add onions and mushrooms and cook for 5 minutes. Stir in sour cream, salt, and pepper.

3 Transfer to a 9" × 13" baking dish. Sprinkle cheese on top.

4 Bake for 20 minutes or until bubbly and golden brown. Allow to cool slightly and serve hot.

Twice-Baked Cauliflower

This Twice-Baked Cauliflower gives the same satisfaction as twice-baked potatoes, but with significantly fewer carbohydrates. The cream cheese thickens the cauliflower so it can hold its shape.

1 large head cauliflower, roughly chopped

1 cup water

1 cup shredded Cheddar cheese, divided

6 slices cooked no-sugar-added bacon, chopped

4 ounces cream cheese

½ cup sour cream

4 green onions, finely chopped

3 tablespoons grass-fed butter

½ teaspoon sea salt

¼ teaspoon ground black pepper

SERVES 6	
Per Serving:	
Calories	299
Fat	26g
Protein	11g
Sodium	565mg
Fiber	2g
Carbohydrates	7g
Net Carbs	5g
Sugar	3g

1 Preheat oven to 350°F.

2 Combine cauliflower and water in a large saucepan and bring to a boil over medium-high heat. Cook until tender, about 5 minutes. Drain and transfer cauliflower to a large bowl.

3 Mash cauliflower with a potato masher. Add ½ cup Cheddar cheese, bacon, cream cheese, sour cream, green onions, butter, salt, and pepper. Mash until butter is melted and ingredients are combined.

4 Transfer mixture to an 8" × 8" baking dish and sprinkle remaining cheese on top. Bake for 30 minutes or until hot and bubbly. Allow to cool slightly, then serve hot.

Garlic-Roasted Radishes

SERVES 6

Per Serving:

Calories	55
Fat	4g
Protein	1g
Sodium	202mg
Fiber	1g
Carbohydrates	3g
Net Carbs	2g
Sugar	2g

RADISHES: THE NON-STARCHY ROOT VEGETABLE

Unlike potatoes, which are loaded with starch, radishes are virtually starch-free. Half of the carbohydrates in radishes come from natural sugars, while the other half come from fiber. Because of this, radishes are low in net carbohydrates, containing only 2 grams of net carbs per cup.

Like turnips, radishes make a great substitute for potatoes when you're following a keto diet. While you can eat them raw in salads, roasting them diminishes their spicy "bite" and brings out a milder, neutral flavor.

3 teaspoons minced garlic

2 tablespoons grass-fed butter, melted

½ teaspoon ground thyme

4 cups radishes, trimmed and halved

½ teaspoon sea salt

¼ teaspoon ground black pepper

2 tablespoons lemon juice

1 Preheat oven to 450°F. Line a baking sheet with parchment paper.

2 Whisk together garlic, butter, and thyme in a medium mixing bowl. Add radishes and toss to coat.

3 Arrange radishes on prepared baking sheet and sprinkle with salt and pepper.

4 Bake for 20 minutes or until tender, turning radishes halfway through cooking. Remove from oven and drizzle lemon juice on top.

5 Serve immediately.

Parmesan Herb Cauliflower

Herbes de Provence usually contain rosemary, fennel, summer savory, thyme, basil, marjoram, lavender, parsley, oregano, and tarragon.

3 tablespoons grass-fed butter, melted

1 teaspoon sea salt

½ teaspoon ground black pepper

1 teaspoon herbes de Provence

1 large head cauliflower, cut into florets

⅓ cup grated Parmesan cheese

SERVES 6	
Per Serving:	
Calories	96
Fat	8g
Protein	4g
Sodium	465mg
Fiber	2g
Carbohydrates	4g
Net Carbs	2g
Sugar	1g

1 Preheat oven to 450°F. Line a baking sheet with parchment paper.

2 Whisk butter, salt, pepper, and herbs in a large mixing bowl. Add cauliflower and toss to coat.

3 Arrange cauliflower in a single layer on prepared baking sheet. Sprinkle Parmesan cheese on top. Bake for 12 minutes or until cauliflower is crisp. Remove from oven and serve hot.

Cilantro Lime Cauliflower Rice

Cilantro and lime add a bright taste to riced cauliflower. If you don't have fresh cilantro, you can use 1⅓ tablespoons dried cilantro.

2 tablespoons olive oil

1 teaspoon minced garlic

1 (12-ounce) bag riced cauliflower

¼ cup chopped fresh cilantro

2 tablespoons fresh lime juice

½ teaspoon granulated onion

½ teaspoon onion salt

¼ teaspoon sea salt

¼ teaspoon ground black pepper

SERVES 6	
Per Serving:	
Calories	58
Fat	5g
Protein	1g
Sodium	250mg
Fiber	1g
Carbohydrates	3g
Net Carbs	2g
Sugar	1g

1 Heat oil in a medium skillet over medium heat. Add garlic and cook for 1 minute. Stir in cauliflower and sauté for 4 minutes. Cover and cook until cauliflower is tender, about 5 minutes.

2 Remove from heat and stir in remaining ingredients. Serve hot.

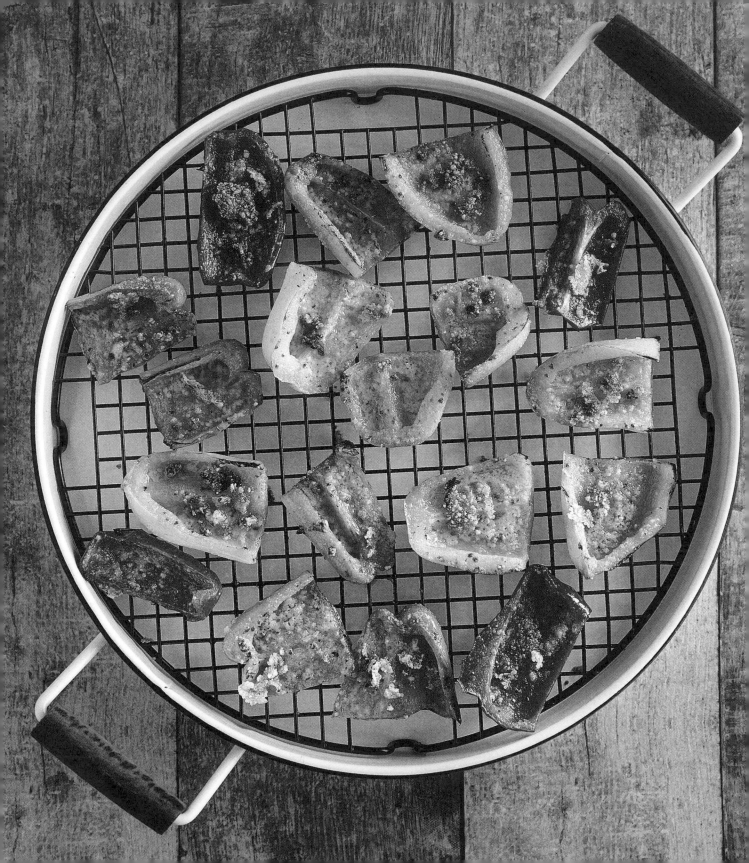

Parmesan-Roasted Mini Sweet Peppers

Mini sweet peppers are slightly higher in carbohydrates than regular bell peppers. If the sweet peppers don't fit into your specific keto plan, you can swap them out with slices of bell peppers instead.

1 pound mini sweet peppers

2 tablespoons olive oil

1 teaspoon sea salt

½ teaspoon ground black pepper

1 teaspoon Italian seasoning

½ teaspoon granulated garlic

¼ cup grated Parmesan cheese

1 Place an oven rack on the highest position and preheat oven broiler to high. Line a baking sheet with parchment paper.

2 Cut the stems off peppers and cut in half lengthwise. Remove seeds and membranes.

3 Whisk olive oil, salt, pepper, Italian seasoning, and garlic together in a medium bowl. Add peppers to bowl and toss to coat.

4 Arrange peppers in a single layer on baking sheet. Sprinkle Parmesan cheese on top and broil for 2 minutes. Flip peppers over and broil for another 2 to 3 minutes or until they just start to look charred.

5 Serve immediately.

SERVES 6	
Per Serving:	
Calories	85
Fat	6g
Protein	3g
Sodium	421mg
Fiber	2g
Carbohydrates	5g
Net Carbs	3g
Sugar	3g

WAYS TO USE MINI SWEET PEPPERS

Roasting mini sweet peppers brings out their natural sweetness, but that's not the only way to eat them. You can slice them in half and use them as a base for stuffed peppers, you can panfry them in oil, you can turn them into a pepper hummus, or you can just eat them straight out of the bag. At only 6 grams of net carbohydrates per cup, they make a great low-carb-day snack.

Thyme Cauliflower Rice with Feta

Per Serving:

Calories	66
Fat	3g
Protein	3g
Sodium	248mg
Fiber	2g
Carbohydrates	6g
Net Carbs	4g
Sugar	3g

IT'S ABOUT THYME

Need a happiness boost? Try thyme! Research shows that regularly eating thyme may help improve both dopamine and serotonin, two neurotransmitters that are essential to a good mood. Thyme may also help fight cancer and boost the immune system, staving off chronic infections like bronchitis.

Thyme belongs to the mint family yet has a very distinctive taste. There's no substitute that matches its flavor profile exactly, but if you don't have it, you can use basil or oregano and still end up with a delicious side dish.

1 tablespoon olive oil

1 cup sliced baby bella mushrooms

1 medium yellow onion, peeled and finely diced

1 cup chopped spinach

2 teaspoons minced garlic

1 (12-ounce) bag frozen riced cauliflower

½ teaspoon sea salt

¼ teaspoon ground black pepper

¼ cup chicken bone broth

2 tablespoons fresh thyme

¼ cup crumbled feta cheese

1 Heat olive oil in a large skillet over medium heat. Add mushrooms and onions and cook for 3 minutes. Add spinach and cook until wilted, about 2 minutes.

2 Stir in garlic, cauliflower, salt, and pepper and cook for 5 minutes.

3 Pour in broth and add thyme. Cook until cauliflower is tender and liquid is absorbed, about 5 minutes. Stir in feta cheese and remove from heat.

4 Serve immediately.

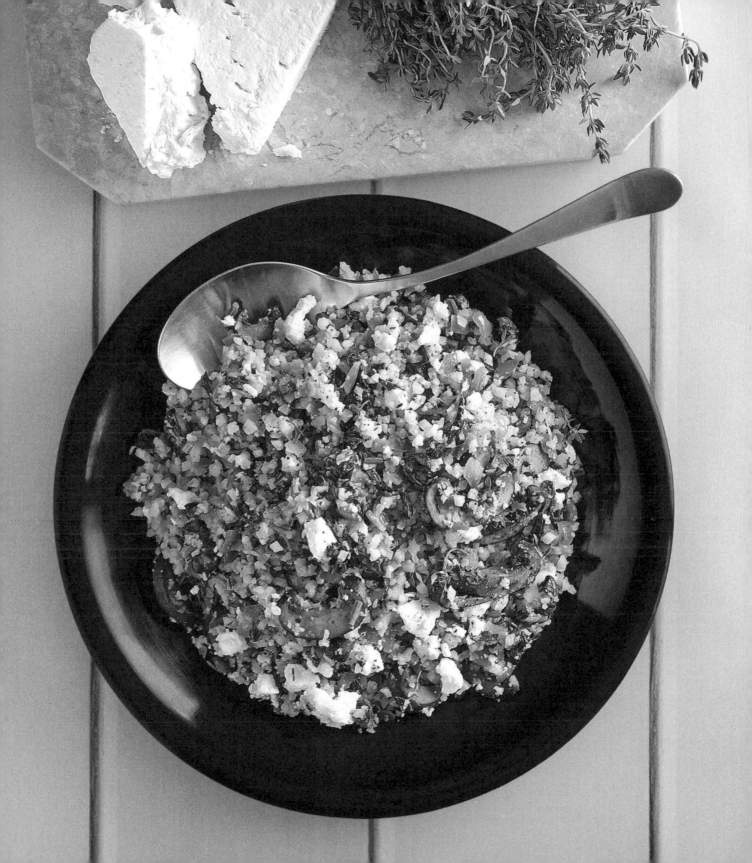

Herb-Roasted Turnips

SERVES 6	
Per Serving:	
Calories	69
Fat	6g
Protein	1g
Sodium	385mg
Fiber	1g
Carbohydrates	4g
Net Carbs	3g
Sugar	2g

Missing potatoes in your keto lifestyle? Try these turnips instead! This root vegetable has a taste and texture similar to white potatoes but with significantly fewer carbs.

3 tablespoons grass-fed butter, melted

1 tablespoon herbes de Provence

2 large turnips, peeled and cubed

1 teaspoon sea salt

1 Preheat oven to 400°F. Line a baking sheet with parchment paper.

2 Whisk together melted butter and herbs in a medium mixing bowl. Add cubed turnips and toss to coat.

3 Arrange turnips in a single layer on prepared baking sheet. Sprinkle with salt. Bake for 30 minutes or until tender. Serve immediately.

Keto Slaw

SERVES 6	
Per Serving:	
Calories	100
Fat	9g
Protein	1g
Sodium	564mg
Fiber	1g
Carbohydrates	7g
Net Carbs	2g
Sugar	2g

Keto Slaw is a quick and easy way to add some healthy fats to any dish. It goes great on top of burgers, alongside roasted chicken, and in your Mason jar salads.

2 tablespoons Dijon mustard

⅓ cup mayonnaise

¼ cup apple cider vinegar

2 tablespoons granulated erythritol

¼ teaspoon ground black pepper

1 teaspoon sea salt

4 cups shredded cabbage

1 Combine mustard, mayonnaise, vinegar, erythritol, pepper, and salt in a medium mixing bowl and whisk together.

2 Add cabbage and toss to evenly coat. Refrigerate for 1 hour before serving.

Spaghetti Squash au Gratin

Au gratin *is a French term that refers to a dish with a browned topping. That could mean covered with bread crumbs or grated cheese and baked. This Spaghetti Squash au Gratin combines the best of both worlds for keto cyclers—low-carb and cheese.*

1 large spaghetti squash

3 tablespoons grass-fed butter

1 teaspoon minced garlic

1 small yellow onion, peeled and sliced into thin strips

½ teaspoon crushed red pepper

½ teaspoon granulated garlic

½ teaspoon sea salt

¼ teaspoon ground black pepper

¾ cup sour cream

1 cup shredded white Cheddar cheese, divided

SERVES 6	
Per Serving:	
Calories	222
Fat	17g
Protein	7g
Sodium	323mg
Fiber	2g
Carbohydrates	11g
Net Carbs	9g
Sugar	4g

1 Preheat oven to 425°F.

2 Carefully cut squash in half lengthwise and scoop out seeds. Place facedown on a baking sheet lined with parchment paper and bake for 45 minutes or until tender.

3 While spaghetti squash is cooking, heat butter in a medium skillet over medium heat. Add minced garlic and onions and cook for 3 minutes. Set aside.

4 Allow spaghetti squash to cool slightly and then remove strands from skin with a fork. Transfer cooked spaghetti squash to a 9" × 13" baking dish. Stir in onion mixture, spices, sour cream, and ½ cup of cheese. Sprinkle remaining cheese on top.

5 Bake for 20 minutes and then turn oven to broil and broil for 3 minutes or until cheese turns golden brown. Remove from oven and allow to cool slightly. Serve hot.

Baked Turnips

SERVES 6

Per Serving:

Calories	79
Fat	4g
Protein	1g
Sodium	421mg
Fiber	2g
Carbohydrates	9g
Net Carbs	7g
Sugar	5g

TURNIPS VERSUS POTATOES

One-half cup of cubed white potatoes contains 13 grams of carbohydrates, while the same quantity of turnips contains only 4.2 grams. Although they're a member of the cabbage family, turnips taste similar to potatoes. As a general rule, the larger the turnip is, the more bitter it will taste, so when choosing turnips, opt for the smaller ones.

Almost 30 percent of the carbohydrates in turnips come from fiber, making the root vegetable fairly low in net carbohydrates. If you want to switch things up for your high-carb day, you can add some sweet potatoes to the dish and bake them all together.

1 tablespoon olive oil

1 tablespoon grass-fed butter

2 teaspoons minced garlic

1 small shallot, peeled and minced

1½ pounds small turnips, peeled, cut in half lengthwise, and cut into half-moons

1 teaspoon sea salt

½ teaspoon ground black pepper

1 tablespoon lemon juice

½ teaspoon lemon zest

3 tablespoons chopped parsley

1 Preheat oven to 400°F.

2 Heat olive oil and butter in a medium skillet over medium heat. Add garlic and shallots and cook for 1 minute. Add turnips, salt, and pepper and cook until browned, about 10 minutes.

3 Transfer to a 9" × 13" baking dish. Bake for 10 minutes. Remove from oven and stir in lemon juice, lemon zest, and parsley. Serve immediately.

CHAPTER 6

Keto Desserts

One-Minute Chocolate Chip Brownie

CACAO VERSUS COCOA

Cacao and cocoa both come from the beans of the cacao plant, but the difference is in their processing. Cacao is cold-pressed, unroasted cacao beans, while cocoa is made by roasting raw cacao at high temperatures. This roasting process not only changes the flavor; it also reduces the enzyme and antioxidant content in the beans. You can use raw cacao powder and cocoa powder interchangeably, but keep in mind that raw cacao is the more nutrient-dense option.

What could be better than a single-serving chocolate chip brownie you make in minutes? If you prefer not to use a microwave, you can mix your ingredients in an oven-safe dish and then bake this brownie in the oven for 12 minutes at 350°F.

2 tablespoons chocolate MCT oil powder

1 tablespoon coconut flour

1 tablespoon granulated monk fruit sweetener

½ teaspoon baking powder

1 tablespoon raw cacao powder

1 large egg

¼ cup unsweetened chocolate almond milk

1 tablespoon grass-fed butter, melted

2 tablespoons stevia-sweetened chocolate chips

1 Combine all ingredients, except chocolate chips, in a microwave-safe mug or ramekin. Stir until smooth.

2 Stir in chocolate chips.

3 Microwave for 50 seconds or until brownie reaches desired doneness.

No-Bake Chocolate Peanut Butter Cookies

These No-Bake Chocolate Peanut Butter Cookies are the go-to choice when you want something sweet but don't want to turn on the oven. They come together in minutes, then just need to sit in the freezer for 1 hour to set.

1⅓ cups no-sugar-added creamy peanut butter

1 teaspoon vanilla extract

2 tablespoons raw cacao powder

2 cups unsweetened coconut flakes

2 tablespoons grass-fed butter, melted

2 tablespoons golden monk fruit sweetener

¼ cup stevia-sweetened chocolate chips

SERVES 8 (MAKES 16 COOKIES)	
Per Serving:	
Calories	402
Fat	38g
Protein	12g
Sodium	92mg
Fiber	5g
Carbohydrates	15g
Net Carbs	5g
Sugar	1g

1 Line a baking sheet with parchment paper.

2 Combine all ingredients in a medium mixing bowl and stir until incorporated.

3 Use a 1.25" cookie scoop to spoon mixture onto prepared baking sheet. Press scooped dough into cookie shapes.

4 Freeze for 1 hour or until set. Remove from parchment paper and transfer to an airtight container. Store in the refrigerator for 2 weeks or in the freezer for up to 2 months until ready to eat.

Brownie Cheesecake

It's always a good idea to try to make your dessert treats as nutrient-dense as possible. The pecans and Greek yogurt in this dish add some protein and important fatty acids. Make sure you're using coconut cream instead of coconut milk for this Brownie Cheesecake. Not only will it give the cheesecake a richer, creamy texture, but it will also boost the fat content.

SERVES 12	
Per Serving:	
Calories	420
Fat	35g
Protein	7g
Sodium	132mg
Fiber	4g
Carbohydrates	30g
Net Carbs	18g
Sugar	15g

BENEFITS OF PECANS

Pecans are rich in manganese and copper—two minerals that boost energy and help you lose weight. Researchers believe that these two nutrients work together to maintain more than fifty different enzyme reactions that keep your metabolism strong and help create adenosine triphosphate (ATP)—the compound that gives you energy. A single 3.5-ounce serving of pecans contains 2 to 2.5 times the amount of manganese you need for the entire day.

1 cup raw pecans

1 tablespoon raw cacao powder

½ teaspoon stevia powder

3 tablespoons grass-fed butter, melted

1 cup coconut cream

1 cup unsweetened baking chocolate

½ cup granulated monk fruit sweetener

2 (8-ounce) packages cream cheese

½ cup full-fat plain Greek yogurt

1 Preheat oven to 300°F.

2 Combine pecans, cacao powder, stevia powder, and melted butter in a food processor and pulse for 1 minute until crumbly.

3 Transfer mixture to a 9" springform pan and press into bottom of pan to form a crust.

4 Heat coconut cream in a medium saucepan over medium heat. When cream is hot, remove from heat and stir in baking chocolate and monk fruit sweetener, whisking constantly until chocolate is melted and mixture is smooth.

5 Combine cream cheese and Greek yogurt in a medium bowl and beat with a handheld mixer on low speed until smooth. Fold cream cheese mixture into chocolate mixture and stir until combined.

6 Pour cream cheese mixture over crust and spread into an even layer. Bake for 90 minutes or until cheesecake sets.

7 Allow to cool completely before serving.

Chocolate Chip Cookie Bake

Chocolate chip cookies are a classic favorite, but sometimes separating the dough into individual cookies can take a lot of extra work and time. This low-carb version allows you to bake the cookies right in a pie plate, so there's no fuss necessary.

½ cup butter-flavored coconut oil

1 large egg

1 teaspoon vanilla extract

3 tablespoons golden monk fruit sweetener

3 tablespoons granulated monk fruit sweetener

2 cups almond flour

½ teaspoon sea salt

½ cup stevia-sweetened chocolate chips

SERVES 8	
Per Serving:	
Calories	342
Fat	31g
Protein	7g
Sodium	137mg
Fiber	4g
Carbohydrates	18g
Net Carbs	4g
Sugar	1g

1 Preheat oven to 350°F.

2 Heat coconut oil in a small skillet over medium-high heat. Bring to a bubble and then reduce heat to low.

3 Cook for 3 minutes or until oil starts to turn golden. Remove from heat and allow to cool slightly.

4 Combine egg, vanilla, and sweeteners in a medium bowl and beat with a handheld mixture until fluffy. Add oil and beat until smooth.

5 Stir in almond flour and salt and mix until just combined. Add chocolate chips and stir to incorporate.

6 Transfer dough to a 9" pie plate and press down mixture evenly into pan.

7 Bake for 25 minutes or until a toothpick inserted in the center comes out clean. Allow to cool slightly before serving.

BAKING WITH ALMOND FLOUR

Almond flour is the basis of many keto recipes because it's one of the most versatile low-carb flours and works well in everything from cookies to cakes to breading for chicken. But not all almond flour is created equally. When baking with almond flour, you generally get the best result by using fine-milled, blanched almond flour, especially in baked goods that require extra care like cake and bread. Coarse almond flour or almond meal is a better option when using it to "bread" chicken or fish.

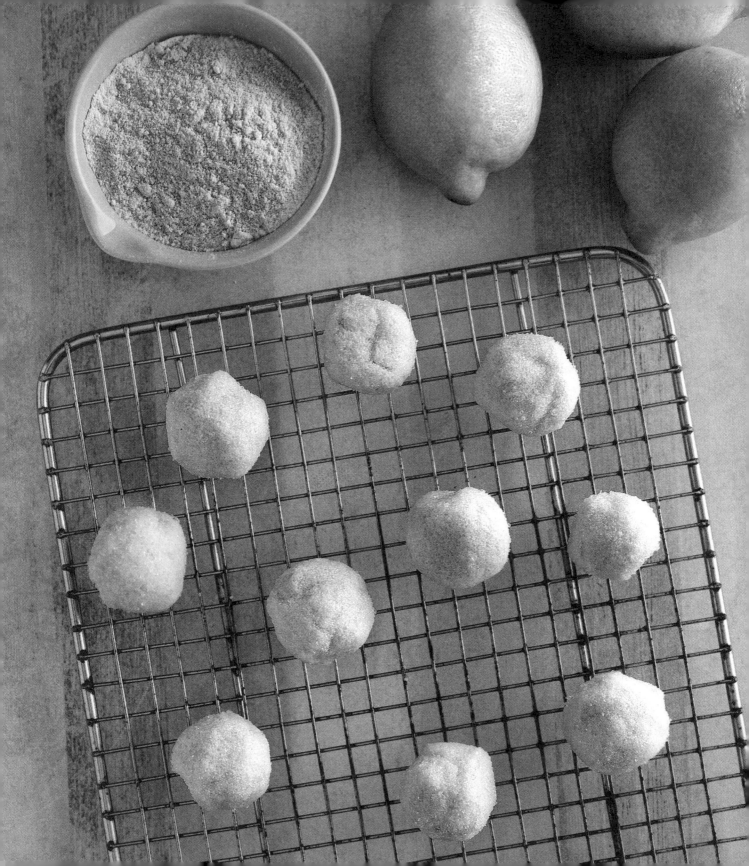

Lemon Coconut Bites

Although bottled lemon juice is keto-friendly, try to stick with fresh-squeezed juice. It not only has a fresher taste; it also still contains all of its nutrients since it's not processed with added preservatives.

¼ cup cream cheese, softened

2 teaspoons lemon juice

1 teaspoon lemon zest

½ cup coarse almond flour

1 tablespoon coconut flour

4 tablespoons granulated erythritol, divided

½ teaspoon vanilla extract

⅛ teaspoon sea salt

SERVES 5 (MAKES 10 BITES)	
Per Serving:	
Calories	105
Fat	9g
Protein	3g
Sodium	91mg
Fiber	2g
Carbohydrates	13g
Net Carbs	1g
Sugar	1g

1 Line a baking sheet with parchment paper.

2 Combine all ingredients, except 2 tablespoons erythritol, in a medium bowl and beat with a handheld mixer until smooth.

3 Use a 1¼" cookie scoop to form balls. Dip balls in remaining erythritol and roll to coat.

4 Arrange balls on prepared baking sheet. Freeze for 1 hour or until set.

5 Transfer balls to an airtight container and store in the refrigerator for up to 2 weeks until ready to eat.

Coconut Butter Cups

These Coconut Butter Cups are rich in medium-chain triglycerides, or MCTs, a specific type of fat that has been shown to keep you full for longer than other types. They're a great choice when you're trying to stave off hunger in between meals.

½ cup raw cacao powder

½ cup butter-flavored coconut oil, melted

8 drops liquid stevia, divided

½ cup coconut butter, melted

1 Line 18 wells of a mini muffin tin with paper or silicone liners.

2 Combine cacao powder, melted coconut oil, and 4 drops of stevia in a medium bowl and stir until smooth. Divide the chocolate mixture in half and pour evenly into each prepared well.

3 Freeze for 30 minutes. Mix remaining stevia with coconut butter and pour mixture evenly on top of each well. Freeze for 30 minutes.

4 Pour remaining cocoa mixture on top of coconut butter and freeze for 30 minutes. Remove coconut butter cups from muffin tin and transfer to an airtight container.

5 Store in the refrigerator for up to 2 weeks or in the freezer for up to 2 months until ready to eat.

SERVES 9 (MAKES 18 CUPS)

Per Serving:

Calories	217
Fat	22g
Protein	2g
Sodium	5mg
Fiber	3g
Carbohydrates	6g
Net Carbs	3g
Sugar	1g

COCONUT, BY ANY OTHER NAME

Coconut oil and coconut butter are two very different products. As the name implies, coconut oil is the extracted oil from the coconut. Coconut butter is made by puréeing coconut meat into a spread, like butter or peanut butter. The two cannot be used interchangeably.

Chocolate Peanut Butter Cups

If you're like most people, you love a good peanut butter cup, but unfortunately, the familiar childhood favorite in the orange wrapper is out for a keto diet (yes, even on high-carb days). These low-carb Chocolate Peanut Butter Cups give you all the delicious flavor without the added sugar.

8 ounces cream cheese, softened

¼ cup powdered erythritol

¼ cup coconut cream

1 teaspoon vanilla extract

¼ cup no-sugar-added creamy peanut butter

2 tablespoons chopped raw peanuts

⅔ cup stevia-sweetened chocolate chips

2 teaspoons butter-flavored coconut oil

SERVES 9 (MAKES 18 CUPS)	
Per Serving:	
Calories	266
Fat	21g
Protein	5g
Sodium	82mg
Fiber	2g
Carbohydrates	24g
Net Carbs	14g
Sugar	6g

1 Line 18 wells of a mini muffin tin with paper or silicone liners.

2 Combine cream cheese, erythritol, and coconut cream in a medium mixing bowl. Beat with a handheld mixer until smooth.

3 Beat in vanilla extract and peanut butter. Stir in peanuts.

4 Combine chocolate chips and coconut oil in a small saucepan. Heat over low heat until melted and smooth.

5 Pour chocolate into each of the prepared muffin wells. Freeze for 30 minutes or until chocolate sets.

6 Scoop peanut butter mixture on top of set chocolate and press with a spoon to form an even layer. Freeze for 30 minutes or until set.

7 Transfer cups from muffin tin to an airtight container and store in the refrigerator for up to 2 weeks or in the freezer for up to 2 months, until ready to eat.

Iced Mocha Pops

These pops are a nice way to cool down and get a little caffeine buzz on a hot day. They're rich in MCTs, so you'll satisfy a chocolate craving while also giving your body the sustained energy it needs.

SERVES 10	
Per Serving:	
Calories	26
Fat	2g
Protein	0g
Sodium	38mg
Fiber	2g
Carbohydrates	4g
Net Carbs	0g
Sugar	0g

1¾ cups strongly brewed coffee

½ cup unsweetened chocolate almond milk

½ cup full-fat coconut milk

½ cup monk fruit–sweetened maple syrup

1 tablespoon raw cacao powder

2 tablespoons chocolate MCT oil powder

1   Combine all ingredients in a medium bowl and beat with a hand-held mixer until powders are dissolved and mixture is smooth.

2   Pour mixture into Popsicle molds and freeze until set, about 12 hours.

3   Store in the freezer for up to 1 month until ready to eat.

Peanut Butter Fudge

The peanut flour really deepens the peanut taste in this decadent fudge, but if you don't have it, you can replace it with an equal amount of almond flour.

SERVES 16	
Per Serving:	
Calories	183
Fat	19g
Protein	2g
Sodium	45mg
Fiber	0g
Carbohydrates	3g
Net Carbs	1g
Sugar	1g

8 ounces cream cheese

1 cup butter-flavored coconut oil

1 cup no-sugar-added creamy peanut butter

1 cup granulated monk fruit sweetener

½ cup peanut flour

1   Line a 9" × 9" baking dish with parchment paper.

2   Combine cream cheese and oil in a medium saucepan and melt over medium heat. Stir until combined. Add peanut butter and stir until smooth. Remove from heat and stir in remaining ingredients.

3   Pour mixture into prepared pan and spread in an even layer. Refrigerate for 4 hours or until set.

Strawberry Cheesecake Pops

If you can't find mascarpone cheese, you can use cream cheese in its place for an equally delicious result. However, the mascarpone cheese has a higher fat content, which also means it has a richer, creamier taste.

1 cup frozen sliced strawberries

½ teaspoon lemon juice

1 (8-ounce) package mascarpone cheese

1 cup full-fat coconut milk

¼ cup granulated erythritol

10 drops liquid stevia

2 teaspoons vanilla extract

1   Place strawberries and lemon juice in a food processor and process until broken down, about 1 minute.

2   Combine remaining ingredients in a medium bowl and beat until smooth. Fold in strawberries and stir until combined.

3   Pour mixture evenly into a six-well Popsicle mold. Freeze for 6 hours or until set.

4   Keep in the freezer for up to 1 month until ready to eat.

SERVES 6	
Per Serving:	
Calories	221
Fat	22g
Protein	4g
Sodium	80mg
Fiber	1g
Carbohydrates	12g
Net Carbs	2g
Sugar	3g

THE FAT IN MASCARPONE

Mascarpone cheese clocks in at a whopping 50 percent fat, which makes it an easy way to sneak in fat grams on a keto diet. It has a texture similar to that of cream cheese—although it's a lot richer and creamier—so you can use it in place of cream cheese in most recipes that call for it. True mascarpone cheese is made by using lactic fermentation, a process that introduces probiotics, which can help boost gut health, and thickens the cream.

Almond Clusters

SERVES 6	
Per Serving:	
Calories	302
Fat	25g
Protein	6g
Sodium	4mg
Fiber	4g
Carbohydrates	16g
Net Carbs	5g
Sugar	1g

These Almond Clusters are simple and delicious, and they don't require any baking. You can enjoy them exactly as written or add in some of your favorite keto-friendly mix-ins, like different nuts, unsweetened coconut flakes, and hemp hearts.

3 tablespoons grass-fed butter

¼ cup heavy cream

2 tablespoons granulated monk fruit sweetener

1 teaspoon vanilla extract

1 cup chopped raw almonds

½ cup stevia-sweetened chocolate chips

1 Line a baking sheet with parchment paper.

2 Heat butter in a small saucepan over medium heat. Whisk constantly, until butter starts to turn golden brown. Reduce heat to low, add cream, sweetener, and vanilla and whisk until smooth.

3 Continue whisking over low heat until mixture thickens, about 5 minutes.

4 Remove from heat and stir in almonds. Add chocolate chips and stir quickly once or twice, just enough to mix in the chips but not make them melt completely.

5 Spoon by tablespoonfuls onto prepared baking sheet. Place baking sheet in the freezer and freeze for 30 minutes. Remove from baking sheet and transfer to an airtight container.

6 Store in the refrigerator for up to 2 weeks or in the freezer for up to 2 months until ready to eat.

Blueberry Vanilla Cupcakes

These Blueberry Vanilla Cupcakes are perfectly sweet without anything on top; but if you want to add a little oomph on top, you can make a quick lemon glaze by whisking together 3 tablespoons of fresh lemon juice and ½ cup powdered erythritol.

2 cups almond flour

2 teaspoons baking powder

1 teaspoon vanilla MCT oil powder

¼ teaspoon sea salt

½ cup butter-flavored coconut oil

¼ cup granulated erythritol

2 teaspoons vanilla extract

4 large eggs

¼ cup water

½ cup frozen wild blueberries

1 Preheat oven to 350°F. Line a muffin tin with paper or silicone liners.

2 Combine almond flour, baking powder, MCT oil powder, and salt in a medium mixing bowl.

3 In a separate medium bowl, combine remaining ingredients, except blueberries, and stir until smooth.

4 Add flour mixture to coconut oil mixture and stir until just combined. Gently stir in blueberries.

5 Pour mixture evenly into each muffin well. Bake for 15 minutes or until a toothpick inserted in the center of a cupcake comes out clean.

6 Remove from oven and allow to cool before serving.

SERVES 12

Per Serving:

Calories	204
Fat	19g
Protein	5g
Sodium	67mg
Fiber	2g
Carbohydrates	8g
Net Carbs	2g
Sugar	1g

CHECK YOUR FREEZER SECTION

Wild blueberries contain two times the antioxidants as conventional blueberries, most of which are found in their skin. Because the wild blueberry season is so short, most of the wild blueberries available for purchase are frozen. The good news? None of the antioxidant value is lost during freezing, and they'll keep in your freezer for up to 2 years!

Raspberry Shortbread Cookies

Per Serving:

Calories	174
Fat	16g
Protein	4g
Sodium	2mg
Fiber	3g
Carbohydrates	14g
Net Carbs	3g
Sugar	1g

QUICK CHIA JAM

Finding unsweetened jams can be difficult. Fortunately, it's easy to make your own at home with just five ingredients. Combine 1¼ cups mashed raspberries, 1 teaspoon lemon juice, 1 tablespoon granulated monk fruit sweetener, and ⅓ cup water in a food processor and process until smooth. Transfer to a glass jar and stir in 3 tablespoons of chia seeds. Cover and refrigerate until jam has set, about 4 hours. You can follow these steps with any of your favorite fruits.

The gooey texture of the raspberry jam pairs nicely with the crunchy sweetness of the shortbread in these Raspberry Shortbread Cookies. If you're not going to eat them all within a week, you can freeze them for up to 2 months and pull them out to thaw when you want to devour them.

2 cups almond flour

½ teaspoon baking powder

½ cup grass-fed butter, softened

½ cup powdered erythritol

1 large egg yolk

1 teaspoon vanilla extract

½ cup unsweetened raspberry jam

1 Preheat oven to 325°F. Line a baking sheet with parchment paper.

2 Combine almond flour and baking powder in a small bowl. Set aside.

3 In a medium bowl, combine butter and erythritol and beat until smooth and fluffy. Beat in egg yolk and vanilla extract.

4 Fold almond flour mixture into butter mixture and stir until just incorporated.

5 Form mixture into 24 1" balls and arrange on prepared baking sheet. Bake for 10 minutes.

6 Remove from oven and immediately use a small spoon to press down in the middle of each cookie to form a well.

7 Scoop 1 teaspoon of raspberry jam into each well. Allow to cool before serving.

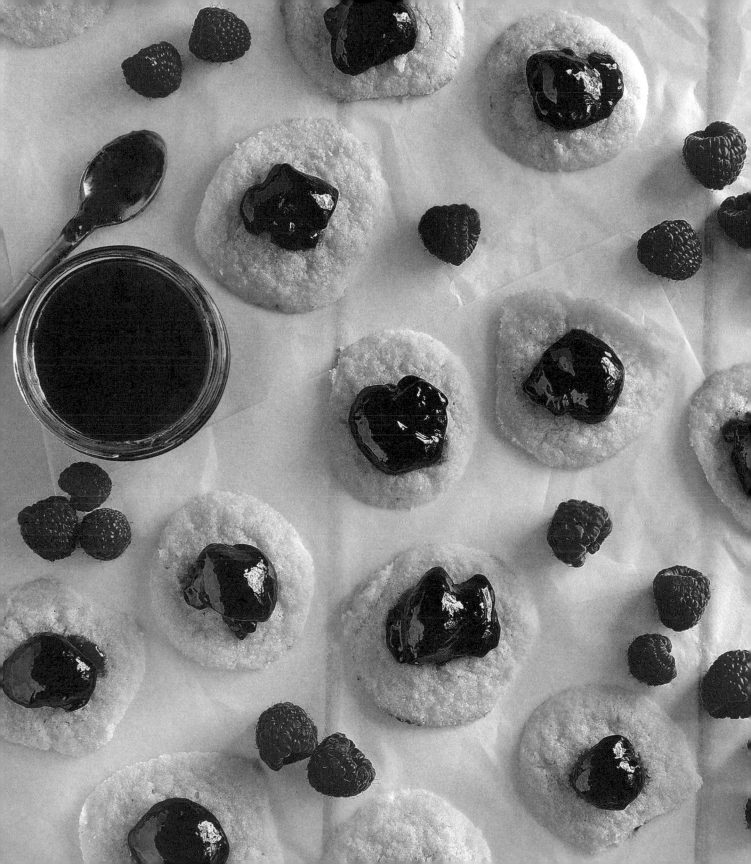

Lemon Cheesecake Mousse

SERVES 4

Per Serving:

Calories	527
Fat	52g
Protein	11g
Sodium	213mg
Fiber	0g
Carbohydrates	22g
Net Carbs	6g
Sugar	5g

PRESERVATIVES IN BOTTLED JUICE

Many bottled juices, including lemon juice, contain a preservative called *sulfur dioxide*, which belongs to a class of preservatives called *sulfites*. Sulfur dioxide has been linked to breathing troubles and asthma-like symptoms. Whenever you can, try to use fresh lemon juice (and other juices) in your recipes to avoid added preservatives and reap the full health benefits of the lemon.

This Lemon Cheesecake Mousse is rich and creamy, while also somehow being light and airy as well. The fresh lemon juice brightens up the flavor and offsets the heaviness of the fat nicely.

8 ounces cream cheese, softened
1 teaspoon vanilla extract
1½ cups heavy whipping cream
1 teaspoon lemon zest
2 tablespoons lemon juice
⅓ cup granulated erythritol
2 tablespoons grass-fed beef gelatin

1 Beat cream cheese and vanilla in a medium bowl with a handheld mixer until smooth and creamy.

2 Add heavy whipping cream and continue beating until soft peaks form, about 3 minutes.

3 Stir in remaining ingredients. Divide mixture equally into four 8-ounce Mason jars or glass jars with lids.

4 Refrigerate for 4 hours or until set.

5 Store in the refrigerator for up to 1 week until ready to eat.

Peanut Butter Cheesecake Mousse

If you don't eat peanut butter, you can replace it with no-sugar-added almond butter, sunflower seed butter, or cashew butter. The taste will differ slightly, but you'll still end up with a delicious, airy low-carb mousse.

8 ounces cream cheese, softened

1 teaspoon vanilla extract

1½ cups heavy whipping cream

¼ cup powdered peanut butter

⅓ cup granulated erythritol

2 tablespoons grass-fed beef gelatin

1 Beat cream cheese and vanilla in a medium bowl with a handheld mixer until smooth and creamy.

2 Add heavy whipping cream and continue beating until soft peaks form, about 3 minutes.

3 Stir in remaining ingredients. Divide mixture equally into four 8-ounce Mason jars or glass jars with lids.

4 Refrigerate for 4 hours or until set.

5 Store in the refrigerator for up to 2 weeks until ready to eat.

SERVES 4

Per Serving:

Calories	550
Fat	53g
Protein	13g
Sodium	259mg
Fiber	1g
Carbohydrates	24g
Net Carbs	7g
Sugar	5g

GELATIN OR COLLAGEN?

Gelatin and collagen come from the same place (bones of cows or marine animals) and have the same amino acid profile, but the way they're processed makes the way they act in recipes vastly different. Collagen dissolves in both hot and cold liquid without changing the structure. Gelatin dissolves only in hot liquid and turns it into a gel-like substance. Although they can't be used interchangeably, they both have their place, and they both support healthy bones, skin, hair, and joints and help repair your gut lining.

Matcha Mug Cake

Matcha tea is a powerhouse when it comes to nutrition. It supports heart health, boosts metabolism, helps improve mood and focus, and can aid in detoxification. Make sure to whisk the almond milk and matcha together until the matcha powder dissolves completely. If you mix it all in together, you'll have a hard time getting the matcha into the rest of the ingredients smoothly.

SERVES 1

Per Serving:

Calories	272
Fat	23g
Protein	8g
Sodium	485mg
Fiber	4g
Carbohydrates	8g
Net Carbs	0g
Sugar	1g

1 tablespoon unsweetened vanilla almond milk

½ teaspoon matcha powder

1 large egg

1 tablespoon granulated monk fruit sweetener

2 teaspoons vanilla MCT oil powder

1 tablespoon grass-fed butter, melted

1 tablespoon coconut flour

¼ teaspoon baking powder

⅛ teaspoon sea salt

1 Combine almond milk and matcha powder in a microwave-safe mug and whisk until smooth.

2 Add egg and whisk until combined.

3 Stir in remaining ingredients.

4 Microwave for 60 seconds and check for doneness by inserting a toothpick in the center of the cake. It's done if the toothpick comes out clean. If cake isn't set, microwave in 15-second intervals until set. Allow to cool slightly before serving.

Peanut Butter Chocolate Chip Blondies

Peanut flour is sold in light and dark roast varieties. Light roast peanut flours have a milder flavor, whereas dark roast flours have a deeper peanut butter flavor. If you're looking for a big peanut pay-off, opt for the darker roast flour.

½ cup grass-fed butter, melted

¾ cup golden monk fruit sweetener

½ cup no-sugar-added creamy peanut butter

2 large eggs

1½ teaspoons vanilla extract

1 cup almond flour

⅓ cup peanut flour

½ teaspoon sea salt

½ cup stevia-sweetened chocolate chips

SERVES 12	
Per Serving:	
Calories	252
Fat	21g
Protein	6g
Sodium	99mg
Fiber	3g
Carbohydrates	22g
Net Carbs	7g
Sugar	1g

1 Preheat oven to 350°F.

2 Combine butter, monk fruit sweetener, and peanut butter in a medium bowl and beat until smooth.

3 Whisk in eggs and vanilla extract.

4 In a small bowl, combine almond flour, peanut flour, and salt. Fold into peanut butter mixture and stir until just incorporated. Stir in chocolate chips.

5 Transfer batter to a 9" × 9" baking pan and spread out evenly.

6 Bake for 20 minutes or until a toothpick inserted in the center comes out clean. Remove from heat and allow to cool before serving.

Chocolate Chip Pumpkin Bars

SERVES 12

Per Serving:

Calories	162
Fat	12g
Protein	3g
Sodium	103mg
Fiber	2g
Carbohydrates	15g
Net Carbs	5g
Sugar	1g

IS PUMPKIN OKAY FOR LOW-CARB DAYS?

Although pumpkin isn't classified as a low-carb vegetable, you can successfully incorporate it into your keto lifestyle, even on low-carb days. Most keto-friendly recipes that use pumpkin purée use a small enough amount that the added carbohydrates don't significantly affect each serving. In larger amounts, pumpkin is a great high-starch vegetable to boost your carbohydrates on high-carb days. Either way, make sure you're using pumpkin purée and not pumpkin pie filling!

Make sure you're using pumpkin purée and not pumpkin pie filling for this recipe. Although the cans look the same, pumpkin pie filling contains added sugars that will quickly kick you out of ketosis.

½ cup grass-fed butter, softened
¼ cup golden monk fruit sweetener
¼ cup granulated monk fruit sweetener
1 large egg
1 teaspoon vanilla extract
½ cup pumpkin purée
1 cup paleo flour
½ teaspoon baking soda
¼ teaspoon sea salt
1½ teaspoons pumpkin pie spice
½ cup stevia-sweetened chocolate chips

1 Preheat oven to 350°F. Grease a 9" × 9" baking dish with coconut oil spray.

2 Combine butter and sweeteners in a medium bowl and beat until smooth. Beat in egg and vanilla. Add pumpkin and beat until smooth.

3 In a separate medium bowl, combine flour, baking soda, salt, and pumpkin pie spice. Fold dry ingredients into butter mixture and stir until just combined. Stir in chocolate chips.

4 Transfer mixture to prepared baking dish and spread out evenly.

5 Bake for 22 minutes or until a toothpick inserted in the center comes out clean. Allow to cool slightly before serving.

Sugared Coconut Cookies

Since these Sugared Coconut Cookies don't have any eggs, you can make them no-bake cookies by shaping them into balls and then freezing them for an hour or until set.

2 cups unsweetened shredded coconut

¼ cup granulated monk fruit sweetener, divided

¼ cup unsweetened vanilla almond milk

1 tablespoon cream cheese

¼ teaspoon vanilla extract

1 Preheat oven to 350°F. Line a baking sheet with parchment paper.

2 Place shredded coconut in a food processor and pulse for 1 minute or until coconut forms a fine powder.

3 Add remaining ingredients, reserving 2 tablespoons of sweetener, and pulse until a dough forms.

4 Form dough into 20 balls. Roll each ball in remaining sweetener to coat. Arrange on prepared baking sheet.

5 Bake for 15 minutes or until cookies start to turn slightly golden.

6 Remove from oven and allow to cool slightly before serving.

SERVES 10 (MAKES 20 COOKIES)	
Per Serving:	
Calories	114
Fat	11g
Protein	1g
Sodium	15mg
Fiber	3g
Carbohydrates	4g
Net Carbs	1g
Sugar	1g

Fatty Fudge Pops

SERVES 6	
Per Serving:	
Calories	318
Fat	30g
Protein	6g
Sodium	36mg
Fiber	4g
Carbohydrates	12g
Net Carbs	0g
Sugar	0g

Coconut cream makes these pops extra thick and creamy and adds a welcomed increase in medium-chain triglycerides, or MCTs.

2 cups coconut cream
½ cup unsweetened cocoa powder
⅔ cup granulated monk fruit sweetener

2 large eggs
1 teaspoon vanilla extract
¼ cup unsweetened chocolate almond milk

1 Combine coconut cream, cocoa powder, sweetener, and eggs in a medium saucepan over medium-low heat. Whisk constantly until mixture just reaches a simmer. Remove from heat. Whisk in vanilla extract and almond milk.

2 Pour mixture into a six-well Popsicle mold. Freeze for 6 hours or until set. Store in the freezer until ready to eat, up to 1 month.

Vanilla Matcha Chia Pudding

SERVES 1	
Per Serving:	
Calories	269
Fat	20g
Protein	10g
Sodium	195mg
Fiber	19g
Carbohydrates	22g
Net Carbs	0g
Sugar	2g

Matcha powder contains a small amount of caffeine, but it's not like the caffeine in coffee. Instead of giving you a quick energy spike, matcha provides a sustained energy boost without any jitters or crashes.

3 tablespoons chia seeds
¼ cup full-fat coconut milk
¼ cup unsweetened vanilla almond milk
¼ teaspoon vanilla extract

1 teaspoon vanilla MCT oil powder
¼ teaspoon matcha powder
2 teaspoons granulated monk fruit sweetener

1 Combine all ingredients in a 16-ounce Mason jar (or another type of glass jar with a lid).

2 Shake vigorously and refrigerate for 4 hours or until pudding has set. Serve cold.

Chocolate Cheesecake Mousse

Adding a small amount of instant coffee granules to a chocolate recipe helps enhance the chocolate flavor without adding a coffee taste. If you don't have instant coffee granules, you can omit them from the recipe.

6 tablespoons cream cheese, softened

2 tablespoons grass-fed butter, softened

1 teaspoon vanilla extract

3 tablespoons powdered erythritol

¼ cup unsweetened cocoa powder

½ teaspoon instant coffee granules

3 tablespoons full-fat plain Greek yogurt

1 Combine cream cheese and butter in a medium mixing bowl. Beat with a handheld mixer until light and fluffy, about 1 minute. Add vanilla, erythritol, cocoa powder, and coffee granules and beat until smooth.

2 In a separate medium bowl, beat Greek yogurt for 2 minutes, until light and fluffy. Fold yogurt into cream cheese mixture and stir until just combined.

3 Divide mixture evenly into two glass bowls. Refrigerate for 2 hours or until set. Serve cold.

SERVES 2	
Per Serving:	
Calories	337
Fat	29g
Protein	7g
Sodium	149mg
Fiber	4g
Carbohydrates	35g
Net Carbs	13g
Sugar	4g

POWDERED VERSUS GRANULATED ERYTHRITOL

Powdered erythritol and granulated erythritol are comparable to powdered sugar and granulated sugar, respectively. The powdered erythritol is a finer version of the sweetener that tends to incorporate better into recipes, but you can use them interchangeably. You can also make powdered erythritol from granulated by putting the amount you need into a coffee grinder and grinding it until a light powder forms.

Strawberries and Cream Milkshake

SERVES 1

Per Serving:

Calories	322
Fat	22g
Protein	17g
Sodium	140mg
Fiber	2g
Carbohydrates	27g
Net Carbs	16g
Sugar	11g

The frozen strawberries in this recipe chill the milkshake, but if you want a thicker, creamier consistency, you can freeze the Greek yogurt or coconut milk before using it too.

½ cup full-fat plain Greek yogurt

½ cup full-fat coconut milk

1 tablespoon cream cheese, softened

1 teaspoon vanilla extract

¼ cup frozen sliced strawberries

1 tablespoon vanilla MCT oil powder

1 tablespoon grass-fed collagen powder

Combine all ingredients in a blender and blend until smooth. Serve immediately.

Orange Cream Pops

SERVES 6

Per Serving:

Calories	25
Fat	1g
Protein	0g
Sodium	92mg
Fiber	0g
Carbohydrates	10g
Net Carbs	10g
Sugar	3g

The orange extract in this recipe adds a boost of orange flavor, but if you don't have any, you can simply omit it without negatively affecting the recipe. You can add a touch more orange juice if your carbohydrate allotment allows.

2¾ cups full-fat coconut milk

¾ cup fresh-squeezed orange juice

1 tablespoon orange zest

¼ teaspoon sea salt

½ teaspoon vanilla extract

⅛ teaspoon orange extract

1 Combine ingredients in a blender and blend until smooth.

2 Pour equal parts of mixture into each well of a six-well Popsicle mold.

3 Freeze for 6 hours or until set. Store in the freezer until ready to eat, up to 1 month.

Chocolate Chip Cheesecake Truffles

These Chocolate Chip Cheesecake Truffles are a dessert and a fat bomb all in one. You can eat them as a sweet treat after dinner or incorporate them during the day to help stave off hunger between meals.

¼ cup cream cheese, softened

½ cup almond flour

4 teaspoons granulated monk fruit sweetener

¼ teaspoon vanilla extract

⅛ teaspoon almond extract

¹⁄₁₆ teaspoon sea salt

¼ cup plus 2 tablespoons stevia-sweetened chocolate chips, divided

1½ teaspoons butter-flavored coconut oil

1 Line a baking sheet with parchment paper.

2 Combine cream cheese, almond flour, monk fruit sweetener, vanilla extract, almond extract, and salt in a medium bowl and beat until incorporated. Stir in 2 tablespoons chocolate chips.

3 Divide mixture into ten equal-sized portions and roll each portion into a ball and arrange on prepared baking sheet. Freeze for 10 minutes.

4 While balls are chilling, combine remaining chocolate chips and coconut oil in a small saucepan over low heat. Stir until melted and smooth. Remove from heat.

5 Remove balls from freezer and use a fork to dip into melted chocolate. Transfer coated balls back to baking sheet.

6 Return to freezer until chocolate is set, about 30 minutes. Transfer to an airtight container and store in the refrigerator for up to 2 weeks or in the freezer for up to 2 months, until ready to eat.

**SERVES 5
(MAKES 10 TRUFFLES)**

Per Serving:

Calories	214
Fat	17g
Protein	4g
Sodium	73mg
Fiber	2g
Carbohydrates	15g
Net Carbs	7g
Sugar	2g

POTENCY OF ALMOND EXTRACT

Almond extract is a lot more concentrated than vanilla extract, so a little goes a long way. When using almond extract, you typically need only ⅛ to ¼ teaspoon to give your recipes a strong almond flavor. If you're using almond extract in place of vanilla extract, you need to use only about half of the amount the recipe calls for.

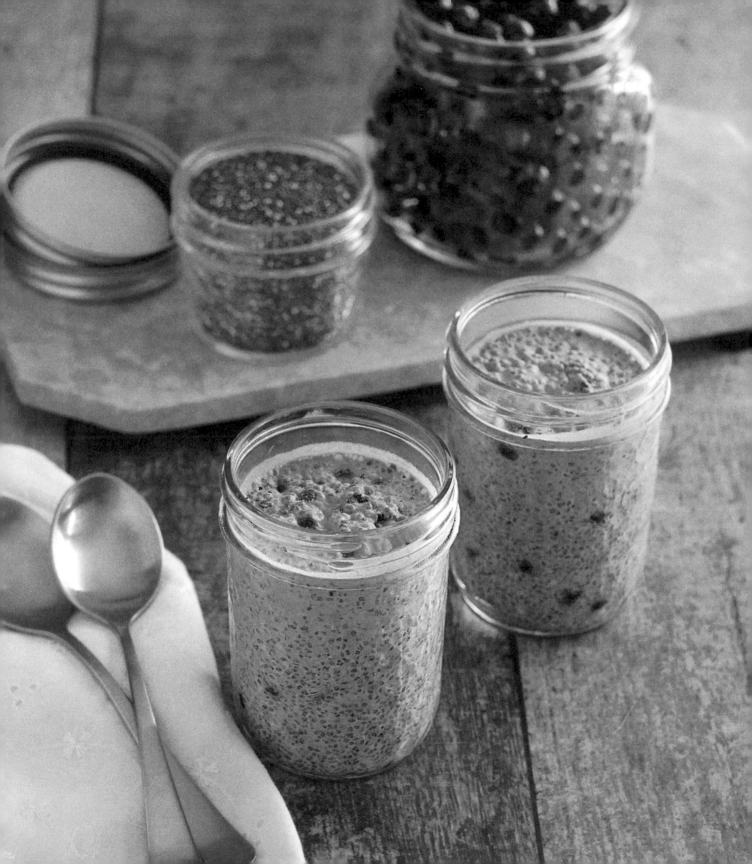

Wild Blueberry Vanilla Chia Pudding

Chia seeds absorb moisture, so the longer they sit in a liquid, the thicker the pudding will get. If you don't eat this pudding right away, you can thin it out to your desired consistency by drizzling in a little extra almond milk.

3 tablespoons chia seeds

¼ cup full-fat coconut milk

¼ cup unsweetened vanilla almond milk

¼ cup frozen wild blueberries

¼ teaspoon vanilla extract

1 teaspoon vanilla MCT oil powder

2 teaspoons granulated monk fruit sweetener

1 Combine all ingredients in two 16-ounce Mason jars (or another type of glass jar with a lid).

2 Shake vigorously and refrigerate for 4 hours or until pudding has set. Serve cold.

SERVES 2	
Per Serving:	
Calories	144
Fat	10g
Protein	5g
Sodium	98mg
Fiber	10g
Carbohydrates	13g
Net Carbs	1g
Sugar	2g

BIG BENEFITS IN A TINY PACKAGE

Almost all of the carbohydrates in chia seeds are in the form of fiber, which contributes to weight loss by absorbing water and expanding in your gut. This helps delay the emptying of your stomach, which means you feel fuller for a longer period of time. A single ounce of chia seeds contains 10 grams of fiber—which is about one-third to one-half the recommended amount for an entire day, depending on if you're a man or a woman. Chia seeds are also rich in protein and essential amino acids.

Strawberry Ice Cream

You can make this decadent ice cream even without an ice cream maker! Simply use the freeze-and-stir method instead. Pour your mixture into a stainless steel baking dish and freeze for 45 minutes. Stir, then return to freezer, stirring every 30 minutes until it reaches desired consistency.

1½ cups frozen whole strawberries

¾ cup granulated monk fruit sweetener

1 tablespoon lemon juice

2 (13.5-ounce) cans full-fat coconut milk

½ teaspoon vanilla extract

1 Combine strawberries, sweetener, and lemon juice in a small saucepan over low heat. Stir, crushing strawberries down with a spoon, until mixture begins to break down and juices are released, about 5 minutes.

2 Remove from heat and allow to cool.

3 Combine strawberry mixture, coconut milk, and vanilla extract in a blender and blend until smooth.

4 Transfer mixture to ice cream maker and process according to manufacturer's instructions.

5 Remove from ice cream maker and transfer to an airtight container. Store in the freezer for up to 2 weeks until ready to eat.

CHAPTER 7

Fat Bombs

Chocolate Brownie Bites

Per Serving:

Calories	75
Fat	8g
Protein	1g
Sodium	1mg
Fiber	1g
Carbohydrates	7g
Net Carbs	0g
Sugar	0g

These decadent treats use high-quality ingredients but should still just be once-in-a-while indulgences. If you prefer your brownies nut-free, you can replace the walnuts with shredded coconut or leave them out completely.

6 tablespoons almond flour

2 tablespoons raw cacao powder

6 tablespoons powdered erythritol

5 tablespoons grass-fed butter, softened

1 teaspoon vanilla extract

3 tablespoons crushed walnuts

1 Line a baking sheet with parchment paper.

2 Combine all ingredients in a small bowl and mix with your hands until fully incorporated. Place bowl in freezer for 15 minutes or until dough firms slightly.

3 Divide dough into 12 equal portions and roll each portion into a ball. Transfer to baking sheet and refrigerate for 1 hour.

4 Transfer brownie bites to an airtight container and store in the refrigerator until ready to eat, up to 1 week.

Pecan Snowball Cookie Bites

There are many keto-friendly maple-flavored syrups that use artificial sweeteners in place of sugar. While these syrups don't have any carbohydrates, artificial sweeteners aren't the ideal choice. Make sure you choose a maple-flavored syrup that's sweetened naturally, instead.

6 tablespoons almond flour

4 tablespoons grass-fed butter, softened

2 tablespoons brown granulated erythritol

1 tablespoon monk fruit–sweetened maple-flavored syrup

3 tablespoons finely chopped pecans

½ teaspoon vanilla extract

2 tablespoons powdered erythritol

1 Line a baking sheet with parchment paper.

2 Combine all ingredients, except powdered erythritol, in a medium bowl and mix with your hands until fully incorporated.

3 Divide dough into 12 equal portions and roll each portion into a ball. Roll each ball in powdered erythritol to coat.

4 Transfer to prepared baking sheet and refrigerate for 1 hour.

5 Transfer to an airtight container and store in the refrigerator until ready to eat, up to 1 week.

SERVES 12	
Per Serving:	
Calories	64
Fat	7g
Protein	1g
Sodium	3mg
Fiber	1g
Carbohydrates	3g
Net Carbs	0g
Sugar	0g

THE DOWNFALLS OF ARTIFICIAL SWEETENERS

Studies show that adults who consume artificial sweeteners tend to take in more calories during the day than adults who don't. What's more, consistently eating artificial sweeteners may trigger the body to make new fat cells. Although the jury is still out, some artificial sweeteners, like aspartame, sucralose, and acesulfame-K, have been linked to cancer.

Everything Bagel Bombs

SERVES 12

Per Serving:

Calories	60
Fat	5g
Protein	1g
Sodium	197mg
Fiber	0g
Carbohydrates	1g
Net Carbs	1g
Sugar	0g

These Everything Bagel Bombs give you all the taste of a toasted everything bagel with cream cheese, but without any of the carbs. They're perfect alongside your morning cup of coffee.

5 ounces cream cheese, softened

1 tablespoon grass-fed butter, softened

1 tablespoon dried chives

2 tablespoons everything bagel seasoning

1 Line a baking sheet with parchment paper.

2 Combine cream cheese and butter in a medium bowl and beat with a handheld mixer until incorporated and fluffy. Stir in chives.

3 Chill in the refrigerator for 1 hour or until mixture firms slightly. Use wet hands to form mixture into 12 balls. Roll each ball in bagel seasoning to lightly coat.

4 Arrange balls on prepared baking sheet and refrigerate for 2 hours. Transfer to an airtight container and refrigerate until ready to eat, up to 1 week.

Peanut Butter Cheesecake Fat Bombs

Peanut butter and cheesecake are a keto dieter's best friends. In this recipe, they're paired together for a fat bomb that's out of this world.

6 tablespoons cream cheese, softened

1 cup full-fat coconut milk

3 tablespoons powdered peanut butter

2 tablespoons granulated erythritol

1 Line an 8" × 8" baking dish with parchment paper.

2 Beat cream cheese in a medium bowl with a handheld mixer until light and fluffy. Add coconut milk and beat until incorporated and smooth.

3 Stir in remaining ingredients.

4 Transfer mixture to prepared baking dish and use a spatula to spread and smooth.

5 Refrigerate overnight.

6 Cut into 12 equal portions and transfer to an airtight container. Store in the refrigerator until ready to eat, up to 1 week.

SERVES 12	
Per Serving:	
Calories	96
Fat	10g
Protein	1g
Sodium	40mg
Fiber	0g
Carbohydrates	3g
Net Carbs	1g
Sugar	1g

Macadamia Chocolate Chip Fat Bombs

SERVES 12	
Per Serving:	
Calories	128
Fat	12g
Protein	2g
Sodium	70mg
Fiber	1g
Carbohydrates	8g
Net Carbs	3g
Sugar	1g

WHAT MAKES MACADAMIA NUTS SO SPECIAL?

Macadamia nuts are higher in fat than other nuts, like almonds, cashews, and walnuts, which makes them an excellent option when you need to add some fat to your meals. More than 75 percent of the fat in macadamia nuts is monounsaturated, the same type of fat that's found in avocados. Studies show that eating foods high in monounsaturated fats can help control blood sugar, even in people with type 2 diabetes.

The macadamia nuts add a deep, rich flavor to these fat bombs, but you can replace them with any nuts that you have on hand without sacrificing any deliciousness.

4 ounces cream cheese, softened

4 tablespoons grass-fed butter, softened

¼ cup no-sugar-added creamy almond butter

3 tablespoons granulated erythritol

¼ teaspoon coarse sea salt

¼ cup stevia-sweetened chocolate chips

2 tablespoons finely chopped macadamia nuts

1 Line a baking sheet with parchment paper.

2 Combine cream cheese and butter in a medium bowl and beat with a handheld mixer until incorporated and fluffy. Beat in almond butter, erythritol, and sea salt. Stir in chocolate chips and macadamia nuts.

3 Divide dough into 12 equal portions and roll each portion into a ball. Transfer to prepared baking sheet.

4 Refrigerate for 2 hours and then transfer to an airtight container. Store in the refrigerator until ready to eat, up to 1 week.

Tiramisu Fat Bombs

Indulge in the distinct flavor of tiramisu with these fat bombs. Espresso is the traditional ingredient in tiramisu, but if you don't have any, you can substitute it with any strongly brewed coffee that you have on hand.

½ cup mascarpone cheese

2 tablespoons grass-fed butter

1 tablespoon MCT oil powder

1 tablespoon raw cacao powder

10 drops liquid stevia

¼ cup brewed espresso

½ teaspoon vanilla extract

½ teaspoon rum extract

1 Line a muffin tin with paper liners.

2 Combine all ingredients in a food processor and process until smooth, about 2 minutes. Pour equal parts of mixture into each prepared muffin well.

3 Freeze for 2 hours or until firm.

4 Remove from muffin tin and transfer to an airtight container. Store in the refrigerator for up to 2 weeks or in the freezer for up to 2 months, until ready to eat.

SERVES 12

Per Serving:

Calories	114
Fat	12g
Protein	1g
Sodium	12mg
Fiber	0g
Carbohydrates	2g
Net Carbs	2g
Sugar	0g

STEVIA VERSUS MONK FRUIT

Stevia and monk fruit are both natural, low-glycemic sweeteners that don't have any calories or carbohydrates. Monk fruit is around 150 to 250 times sweeter than sugar, while stevia is 200 to 400 times sweeter. Although the best keto sweetener depends a lot on personal preference, some people prefer monk fruit because it doesn't have the same bitter aftertaste that many report with stevia. You can use the two interchangeably in any of the recipes that call for them, but make sure to adjust for the different sweetness factor.

Chocolate Caramel Fat Bombs

Make sure to watch this caramel closely as you're cooking it. If you don't stir it enough, it can stick to the bottom of the pan and burn.

SERVES 12

Per Serving:

Calories	242
Fat	24g
Protein	2g
Sodium	84mg
Fiber	1g
Carbohydrates	10g
Net Carbs	4g
Sugar	1g

COCONUT CREAM VERSUS COCONUT MILK

Coconut cream and coconut milk aren't the same thing. Coconut milk has the same consistency as regular milk. It's made from one part coconut and one part water. Coconut cream is much thicker and richer. It's made from four parts coconut and one part water. If you buy a can of coconut milk, the cream typically separates from the rest of the milk. The cream is the thick layer on top and what you should use when recipes call for coconut cream.

10 tablespoons grass-fed butter, softened and divided

¼ cup coconut cream

¼ cup plus 1 tablespoon granulated erythritol, divided

⅛ teaspoon sea salt

6 ounces cream cheese, softened

1 teaspoon vanilla extract

3 tablespoons butter-flavored coconut oil

¼ cup stevia-sweetened chocolate chips

1 Add 4 tablespoons butter to a medium saucepan and melt over medium-high heat. Allow to cook until butter starts to turn golden brown, about 5 minutes. Stir in coconut cream and continue to cook for 3 minutes. Stir in ¼ cup erythritol and salt and continue cooking until mixture cooks down and turns brown, another 4 minutes.

2 Remove mixture from heat and allow to cool slightly. Transfer to a food processor and process until thickened caramel forms. Set aside.

3 Combine remaining butter and cream cheese in a medium mixing bowl. Beat with a handheld mixer until fluffy and incorporated. Beat in vanilla, remaining erythritol, coconut oil, and caramel sauce. Stir in chocolate chips.

4 Divide mixture into 12 equal-sized portions and press each portion into the well of a 1" silicone candy mold. Transfer mold to freezer and chill for 2 hours.

5 Remove fat bombs from mold and transfer to an airtight container. Store in the refrigerator until ready to eat, up to 1 week.

Cinnamon Roll Fat Bombs

Who says you can't have buns of steel and buns of cinnamon? These fat bombs give you all the flavors of a cinnamon roll without throwing you out of ketosis and getting in the way of your fitness goals.

4 ounces cream cheese, softened

4 tablespoons grass-fed butter, softened

¼ cup creamy no-sugar-added sunflower seed butter

¼ cup plus 2 tablespoons granulated erythritol, divided

1½ teaspoons ground cinnamon, divided

1 teaspoon vanilla extract

SERVES 12	
Per Serving:	
Calories	104
Fat	10g
Protein	2g
Sodium	73mg
Fiber	1g
Carbohydrates	8g
Net Carbs	1g
Sugar	1g

1 Line a baking sheet with parchment paper.

2 Combine cream cheese and butter in a medium bowl and beat with a handheld mixer until incorporated and fluffy. Beat in sunflower seed butter, ¼ cup erythritol, 1 teaspoon cinnamon, and vanilla extract until smooth.

3 Refrigerate for 2 hours. Once chilled, divide mixture into 12 equal-sized portions and roll each portion into a ball.

4 Combine remaining erythritol and cinnamon in a small bowl. Roll each fat bomb in erythritol mixture until coated and arrange on prepared baking sheet.

5 Freeze for 1 hour or until set. Transfer fat bombs to an airtight container and store in the refrigerator until ready to eat, up to 1 week.

Strawberry Vanilla Fat Bombs

SERVES 12

Per Serving:

Calories	38
Fat	4g
Protein	0g
Sodium	0mg
Fiber	0g
Carbohydrates	4g
Net Carbs	1g
Sugar	1g

THE CARB COUNT OF STRAWBERRIES

Strawberries are a popular fruit choice on a keto diet because in comparison to other fruits, they're fairly low in carbohydrates. One cup of whole strawberries contains 11 grams of carbohydrates, 3 of which come from fiber, leaving 9 grams of net carbs. Strawberries are a rich source of antioxidants and can help with regulating blood sugar.

These Strawberry Vanilla Fat Bombs are a little higher in carbs than the other fat bombs. You can save them for your higher-carb days or reduce the amount of strawberries you use to lower those numbers.

¾ cup whole frozen strawberries, thawed at room temperature

3 tablespoons granulated erythritol

3 tablespoons almond flour

3 tablespoons grass-fed butter, softened

1 teaspoon vanilla extract

1 Line a baking sheet with parchment paper.

2 Heat strawberries in a small saucepan over medium heat. Add erythritol and simmer for 10 minutes or until mixture has reduced by half.

3 Transfer strawberry mixture to a food processor and process until smooth, about 2 minutes. Add remaining ingredients and process until incorporated, about 1 minute.

4 Remove mixture from food processor and place into a small bowl. Refrigerate for 1 hour or until mixture firms. Divide into 12 equal portions and roll each portion into a ball.

5 Transfer balls to prepared baking sheet and freeze for 1 hour or until firm. Remove from baking sheet and store in an airtight container in the refrigerator until ready to eat, up to 1 week.

Hot Chocolate Fat Bomb

On a cold day, this Hot Chocolate Fat Bomb is just the thing to get rid of the chill. If you want to make this Hot Chocolate Fat Bomb extra creamy, transfer the mixture to a blender after heating and blend for 30 seconds or until frothy.

3 tablespoons grass-fed butter

2 tablespoons raw cacao powder

1 tablespoon MCT oil powder

2 cups full-fat coconut milk

2 tablespoons granulated erythritol

SERVES 2	
Per Serving:	
Calories	558
Fat	58g
Protein	5g
Sodium	69mg
Fiber	3g
Carbohydrates	20g
Net Carbs	5g
Sugar	4g

1 Heat butter in a small saucepan over medium-low heat. Once melted, stir in cacao powder and MCT oil powder until smooth.

2 Add coconut milk and erythritol and continue to stir until smooth.

3 Pour into two mugs. Serve hot.

Peanut Butter Cookie Dough Fat Bombs

If you don't eat peanut butter, you can replace it with equal amounts of no-sugar-added almond butter or sunflower seed butter.

6 tablespoons grass-fed butter, softened

6 ounces cream cheese, softened

3 tablespoons granulated erythritol

¼ cup almond flour

1 teaspoon vanilla extract

½ cup creamy no-sugar-added peanut butter

SERVES 12	
Per Serving:	
Calories	180
Fat	17g
Protein	4g
Sodium	45mg
Fiber	1g
Carbohydrates	6g
Net Carbs	2g
Sugar	1g

1 Line a baking sheet with parchment paper.

2 Beat butter and cream cheese in a medium mixing bowl with a handheld mixer until fluffy. Add remaining ingredients and beat until smooth. Freeze for 30 minutes or until slightly firm.

3 Divide into 12 portions and roll each portion into a ball. Place balls on prepared baking sheet. Freeze for 1 hour. Remove from freezer and transfer balls to an airtight container. Store in the refrigerator, up to 1 week.

Gingerbread Fat Bombs

SERVES 12

Per Serving:

Calories	150
Fat	15g
Protein	2g
Sodium	31mg
Fiber	1g
Carbohydrates	7g
Net Carbs	2g
Sugar	1g

CLOVE: A POWERHOUSE SPICE

Spices get a lot of attention for the flavors they add to dishes, but they don't get as much love for the health benefits, even though they're extremely powerful. Cloves are antibacterial, anticarcinogenic, and anti-inflammatory. They also aid in digestion by stimulating digestive enzymes that help break down food. Cloves may also help regulate blood sugar by increasing the release of insulin and improving the health of the cells that produce insulin.

Gingerbread isn't just for the holiday season. These perfectly spicy fat bombs are a great addition to your keto menu at any time of the year.

½ **cup grass-fed butter, melted**

1 **cup almond flour**

¼ **cup granulated erythritol**

4 **ounces cream cheese, softened**

2 **teaspoons ground cinnamon**

1 **teaspoon ground ginger**

1 **teaspoon ground nutmeg**

⅛ **teaspoon ground cloves**

1 Line a baking sheet with parchment paper.

2 Combine melted butter, almond flour, and erythritol in a medium bowl and stir until smooth. Set aside.

3 In a separate medium bowl, beat cream cheese until fluffy. Beat in butter mixture, cinnamon, ginger, nutmeg, and cloves.

4 Freeze for 1 hour or until firm. Remove from freezer and divide into 12 equal portions. Roll each portion into a ball and arrange on prepared baking sheet.

5 Refrigerate for 1 hour or until firm. Transfer balls to an airtight container and store in the refrigerator until ready to eat, up to 1 week.

Key Lime Pie Fat Bombs

Key limes aren't the same as regular limes. Try to find pre-bottled key lime juice or key limes, which are smaller than traditional limes, in your produce section to get that traditional tangy flavor.

1 cup raw cashews, soaked overnight

½ cup butter-flavored coconut oil, melted

¼ cup coconut butter

¼ cup key lime juice

1 teaspoon key lime zest

2 teaspoons MCT oil powder

⅛ teaspoon stevia powder

1 Line a baking sheet with parchment paper.

2 Combine all ingredients in a food processor and process until smooth.

3 Remove from food processor and transfer to a medium bowl. Refrigerate for 1 hour.

4 Divide into 12 equal portions and roll each portion into a ball. Arrange balls on prepared baking sheet. Refrigerate for 2 hours or until firm.

5 Transfer to an airtight container and store in the refrigerator until ready to eat, up to 1 week.

SERVES 12

Per Serving:

Calories	175
Fat	17g
Protein	2g
Sodium	5mg
Fiber	1g
Carbohydrates	4g
Net Carbs	3g
Sugar	1g

QUICK-SOAKING METHOD

It's best to soak nuts in cold water on the counter for 4 to 8 hours, but if you need to do some soaking in a pinch, you can use a quick-soak method. Combine nuts with boiling water and soak for 10 minutes. Drain water and use nuts. Keep in mind that this quick-soaking method doesn't neutralize antinutrients, which are compounds that make the nuts harder to digest and absorb, but it will make them softer and easier to blend into sauces.

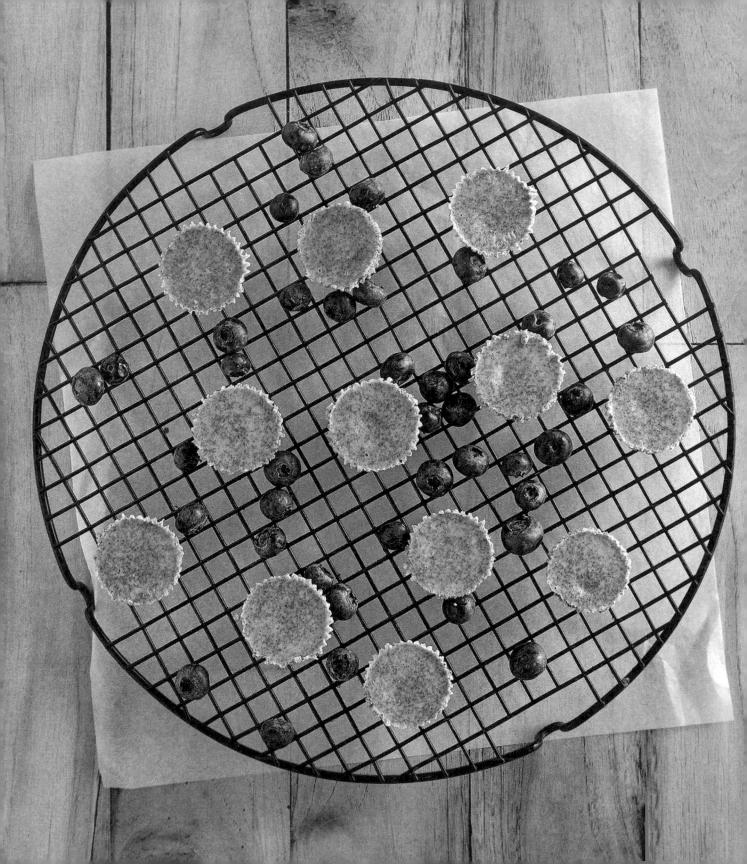

White Chocolate Blueberry Fat Bombs

These unique treats are great if you're a fruit lover. If you can't find freeze-dried blueberries, you can use freeze-dried raspberries, strawberries, blackberries, or a mixture of all of them for this recipe.

¼ **cup freeze-dried wild blueberries**

½ **cup butter-flavored coconut oil**

¼ **cup cacao butter**

¼ **cup powdered erythritol**

1 Line a muffin tin with paper liners.

2 Add blueberries to a food processor and process until a powder forms, about 1 minute. Set aside.

3 Combine coconut oil and cacao butter in a small saucepan and heat over low heat until melted and smooth. Remove from heat.

4 Add blueberry powder and erythritol to coconut oil mixture and stir until smooth.

5 Pour equal amounts of mixture into each prepared muffin well.

6 Refrigerate for 1 hour or until set. Remove fat bombs from muffin tin and transfer to an airtight container.

7 Store in the refrigerator until ready to eat, up to 1 week.

SERVES 12	
Per Serving:	
Calories	122
Fat	14g
Protein	0g
Sodium	0mg
Fiber	0g
Carbohydrates	4g
Net Carbs	1g
Sugar	0g

FREEZE-DRIED FRUIT VERSUS DRIED FRUIT

Freeze-dried fruit and dried fruit are vastly different in texture. Freeze-dried fruit is made by removing 98 to 99 percent of the water from the fruit. The fruit is left with a dry, crunchy texture. Dried fruit is made by removing 90 to 95 percent of the moisture content. The end result is a sticky, chewy fruit. Although you can use small amounts of freeze-dried fruits while on a keto diet, watch your intake. The carbs can add up quickly.

Blueberry Muffin Fat Bombs

Freeze-dried blueberries give these Blueberry Muffin Fat Bombs a nice blueberry flavor without adding too many carbohydrates. If you can't find them, you can add a few dried blueberries to your dough after you take it out of the food processor—but keep an eye on your quantities!

SERVES 12

Per Serving:

Calories	65
Fat	5g
Protein	3g
Sodium	34mg
Fiber	1g
Carbohydrates	4g
Net Carbs	1g
Sugar	1g

3 ounces soft goat cheese

¼ cup freeze-dried blueberries

½ cup almond flour

½ teaspoon vanilla extract

¼ cup almonds

2 tablespoons powdered erythritol

1 Line a baking sheet with parchment paper.

2 Combine all ingredients in a food processor and process until smooth, about 2 minutes.

3 Remove mixture from food processor and divide into 12 equal portions. Roll each portion into a ball and arrange on prepared baking sheet.

4 Refrigerate for 2 hours or until firm. Transfer balls to an airtight container and store in the refrigerator until ready to eat, up to 1 week.

Goat Cheese and Olive Fat Bombs

Who says fat bombs have to be sweet? These savory bites are creamy and salty and can easily help curb a craving in between meals.

4 ounces cream cheese, softened

½ cup crumbled goat cheese

¼ cup grass-fed butter, softened

3 tablespoons chopped fresh basil

6 Kalamata olives, pitted and chopped

2 cloves garlic, minced

¼ teaspoon sea salt

⅛ teaspoon ground black pepper

1 Line a baking sheet with parchment paper.

2 Combine cream cheese, goat cheese, and butter in a medium bowl and beat with a handheld mixer until incorporated and smooth. Stir in remaining ingredients.

3 Refrigerate for 1 hour or until firmed slightly. Divide into 12 equal portions and roll each portion into a ball. Arrange balls on prepared baking sheet.

4 Refrigerate for 2 hours. Transfer balls to an airtight container and store in the refrigerator until ready to eat, up to 1 week.

SERVES 12

Per Serving:

Calories	94
Fat	9g
Protein	2g
Sodium	128mg
Fiber	0g
Carbohydrates	1g
Net Carbs	1g
Sugar	0g

GOAT CHEESE PROTEIN

Cow's milk has two major proteins (whey and casein), but about 80 percent is casein, which can be categorized further into A1 beta-casein and A2 beta-casein. A1 beta-casein is broken down into a compound called *beta-casomorphin-7*, or BCM-7, which has been associated with gastrointestinal inflammation, uncomfortable digestive symptoms, eczema, acne, and cognitive impairment in some people. On the other hand, A2 beta-casein has not been shown to cause any of these ill effects. Goat's milk naturally contains only A2 beta-casein.

Chocolate Fat Bomb Smoothie

SERVES 2	
Per Serving:	
Calories	745
Fat	64g
Protein	25g
Sodium	272mg
Fiber	12g
Carbohydrates	21g
Net Carbs	9g
Sugar	5g

Many grocery stores have frozen avocado available in the frozen fruit section, but if you can't find any, you can cut up fresh avocado and freeze it before making this smoothie; or use it without freezing it for a thinner consistency.

1 cup frozen avocado pieces

2 scoops keto-friendly chocolate protein powder

2 tablespoons cacao powder

2 cups full-fat coconut milk

1 cup ice

1 Combine all ingredients in a blender and blend until smooth.

2 Pour equal amounts into two cups and serve immediately.

Chocolate and Sea Salt Fat Bombs

SERVES 12	
Per Serving:	
Calories	163
Fat	18g
Protein	1g
Sodium	181mg
Fiber	0g
Carbohydrates	2g
Net Carbs	1g
Sugar	0g

If you want to really bring out the flavor in these fat bombs, add a teaspoon of instant coffee granules to deepen the chocolate taste.

½ cup coconut cream

½ cup coconut oil, melted

3 tablespoons grass-fed butter

⅓ cup cream cheese

1 teaspoon vanilla extract

1 teaspoon ground cinnamon

1 teaspoon coarse sea salt

1 tablespoon granulated erythritol

1 Line a muffin tin with paper liners.

2 Combine all ingredients in a food processor and process until smooth. Pour equal amounts of mixture into prepared muffin tin. Refrigerate for 2 hours or until firm.

3 Transfer to an airtight container and store in the refrigerator until ready to eat, up to 1 week.

Cookie Butter Fat Bombs

Unfortunately, that popular cinnamony cookie butter that you can find on store shelves isn't keto-approved, but these fat bombs are.

¼ cup grass-fed butter

2 tablespoons golden monk fruit sweetener

1 tablespoon MCT oil powder

1 teaspoon ground ginger

½ teaspoon ground cinnamon

⅛ teaspoon ground cloves

1 cup no-sugar-added creamy almond butter

SERVES 12	
Per Serving:	
Calories	160
Fat	15g
Protein	5g
Sodium	2mg
Fiber	3g
Carbohydrates	7g
Net Carbs	2g
Sugar	1g

1 Combine all ingredients, except almond butter, in a medium saucepan and heat over medium-low heat until melted. Stir in almond butter. Pour mixture into 12 wells of a silicone candy mold.

2 Freeze for 1 hour. Transfer to an airtight container and store in the refrigerator until ready to eat, up to 1 week.

Golden Milk Fat Bomb Smoothie

You can turn this Golden Milk Fat Bomb Smoothie into a fat bomb latte by omitting the ice and heating all of the ingredients in a saucepan over low heat after blending.

12 ice cubes

3 cups unsweetened vanilla almond milk

2 tablespoons melted coconut oil

¼ cup coconut cream

2 teaspoons vanilla extract

2 tablespoons granulated erythritol

2 tablespoons California Gold Dust Superspice Mix

SERVES 2	
Per Serving:	
Calories	276
Fat	25g
Protein	3g
Sodium	281mg
Fiber	3g
Carbohydrates	34g
Net Carbs	19g
Sugar	1g

1 Combine all ingredients in a blender and blend until smooth.

2 Pour equal amounts into two cups and serve immediately.

Vanilla Matcha Fat Bombs

Matcha is somewhat of an acquired taste, but once you get used to the fresh grassiness, you'll wonder how you ever went so long without it. The vanilla flavoring here adds a mellow complement.

SERVES 12

Per Serving:

Calories	199
Fat	20g
Protein	2g
Sodium	25mg
Fiber	1g
Carbohydrates	7g
Net Carbs	2g
Sugar	1g

CHOOSING YOUR MATCHA

As with coffee, there are different grades of matcha. Ceremonial grade is the highest quality (and most expensive). It's made from the youngest tea leaves and intended to be consumed on its own (only mixed with hot water). Culinary-grade matcha, which is the next step down, is the type most often used in cooking and baking. When using matcha in baked goods, smoothies, and beverages, the culinary grade is your best bet. It has a great flavor profile while still being budget-friendly.

½ **cup coconut oil**

½ **cup coconut butter**

¼ **cup coconut cream**

1 **tablespoon plus 1 teaspoon matcha green tea powder, divided**

⅛ **teaspoon sea salt**

½ **teaspoon vanilla extract**

1 **tablespoon granulated erythritol**

3 **tablespoons powdered erythritol**

1 Line a baking sheet with parchment paper.

2 Combine all ingredients, except 1 teaspoon matcha green tea powder and powdered erythritol, in a food processor and process until smooth.

3 Transfer mixture to a medium bowl and refrigerate for 1 hour or until firm. Combine remaining matcha and powdered erythritol in a small bowl and set aside.

4 Remove balls from refrigerator and divide into 12 equal portions. Roll each portion into a ball and then roll each ball in matcha mixture. Arrange balls on prepared baking sheet. Refrigerate for 2 hours.

5 Transfer balls to an airtight container and store in the refrigerator until ready to eat, up to 1 week.

Chocolate Coffee Fat Bombs

Chocolate and coffee go together like peanut butter and jelly. Although peanut butter and jelly is out in your keto plan, you can satisfy your sweet tooth with these Chocolate Coffee Fat Bombs.

1 cup pecans

1½ tablespoons instant coffee granules

1 teaspoon chocolate MCT oil powder

2 tablespoons raw cacao powder

2 tablespoons granulated erythritol

1 tablespoon butter-flavored coconut oil

½ teaspoon vanilla extract

1 Line a baking sheet with parchment paper.

2 Combine all ingredients in a food processor and process until smooth, about 1 minute.

3 Remove from food processor and divide into 12 equal portions. Roll each portion into a ball and arrange on prepared baking sheet.

4 Refrigerate for 2 hours or until firm. Transfer balls to an airtight container and store in the refrigerator until ready to eat, up to 1 week.

SERVES 12

Per Serving:

Calories	89
Fat	9g
Protein	1g
Sodium	1mg
Fiber	1g
Carbohydrates	4g
Net Carbs	2g
Sugar	0g

HEALTH BENEFITS OF COFFEE

Need a boost in fat burning? Coffee may be able to help. Research shows that caffeine not only boosts your metabolic rate by as much as 3 to 11 percent, but it also increases fat burning directly—up to 10 percent in obese adults and 29 percent in adults at a healthy weight. But don't overdo it! Too much caffeine can increase anxiety and lead to jitters.

Golden Milk Fat Bombs

SERVES 12

Per Serving:

Calories	168
Fat	18g
Protein	1g
Sodium	2mg
Fiber	1g
Carbohydrates	4g
Net Carbs	3g
Sugar	1g

THE PIPERINE IN BLACK PEPPER

To absorb curcumin, which is the compound that gives turmeric all its health benefits, it must be combined with black pepper. This is because black pepper contains a compound called *piperine*, which increases curcumin absorption by 2,000 percent. When making anything with turmeric, always make sure to add a little bit of black pepper or your body won't be able to use it effectively.

If you don't have California Gold Dust powder, you can use a blend of turmeric, cinnamon, ginger, and black pepper in its place. The combination of spices adds an earthy, warming flavor that also helps combat chronic inflammation.

1 cup raw macadamia nuts, soaked overnight
½ cup butter-flavored coconut oil
1 teaspoon vanilla extract
1 tablespoon vanilla MCT oil powder
12 drops liquid stevia
2 teaspoons California Gold Dust Superspice Mix

1 Place macadamia nuts in a food processor and process until smooth, about 2 minutes.

2 Add coconut oil and pulse until smooth, approximately 1 minute.

3 Add remaining ingredients and process until smooth, about 30 seconds.

4 Pour equal amounts of mixture into each well of a silicone candy mold. Freeze for 2 hours.

5 Transfer to an airtight container and store in the refrigerator until ready to eat, up to 1 week.

Cream Cheese Frosting Fat Bombs

The frosting is arguably the best part of any cake. With these Cream Cheese Frosting Fat Bombs, you can have all of that frosting flavor without as many carbs.

4 tablespoons grass-fed butter, softened

4 tablespoons cream cheese, softened

3 tablespoons powdered erythritol

½ teaspoon vanilla extract

⅛ teaspoon sea salt

SERVES 12	
Per Serving:	
Calories	51
Fat	6g
Protein	0g
Sodium	37mg
Fiber	0g
Carbohydrates	3g
Net Carbs	0g
Sugar	0g

1 Combine butter and cream cheese in a medium bowl and beat with a handheld mixer until fluffy and incorporated, about 3 minutes.

2 Add remaining ingredients and beat until smooth.

3 Scoop 12 equal portions into each well of a silicone candy mold and freeze until firm, about 2 hours.

4 Transfer to an airtight container and store in the refrigerator until ready to eat, up to 1 week.

Lemon Tart Fat Bombs

SERVES 12

Per Serving:

Calories	176
Fat	17g
Protein	2g
Sodium	6mg
Fiber	1g
Carbohydrates	7g
Net Carbs	4g
Sugar	1g

ZESTING WITH CARE

When zesting any citrus fruit, always make sure to use a grater made specifically for zesting and turn the fruit as you go. You want to zest the colorful part of the skin and avoid the white part, called the *pith*. Unlike zest from the skin, which has a bright, citrusy flavor, the pith is bitter and will negatively affect the taste of your food.

Don't skip the zest in this recipe! It may seem like a small amount, but adding the zest to the fat bombs really brings out the lemon flavor.

1 cup raw cashews, soaked overnight

½ cup butter-flavored coconut oil, melted

¼ cup coconut butter

2 tablespoons fresh lemon juice

1 teaspoon lemon zest

2 tablespoons coconut flour

2 tablespoons granulated erythritol

1 Line a baking sheet with parchment paper.

2 Combine all ingredients in a food processor and process until smooth, about 1 minute.

3 Transfer to a small bowl and refrigerate for 1 hour. Remove from refrigerator and divide mixture into 12 equal portions. Roll each portion into a ball and arrange on prepared baking sheet.

4 Refrigerate for 2 hours or until firm. Transfer to an airtight container and store in the refrigerator until ready to eat, up to 1 week.

Chocolate Cheesecake Fat Bombs

Chocolate and cheesecake flavors mix perfectly in this treat. The chocolate MCT oil powder in these Chocolate Cheesecake Fat Bombs increases the fat content and deepens the chocolate flavor, but if you don't have it, you can leave it out.

8 ounces cream cheese, softened

½ cup grass-fed butter

¼ cup powdered erythritol

¼ cup raw cacao powder

¼ cup no-sugar-added sunflower seed butter

1 tablespoon chocolate MCT oil powder

1　Line a baking sheet with parchment paper.

2　Combine all ingredients in a food processor and process until smooth, about 1 minute. Transfer mixture to a small bowl and refrigerate for 1 hour.

3　Divide mixture into 12 equal portions and roll each portion into a ball. Arrange on baking sheet.

4　Refrigerate for 2 hours or until firm. Transfer to an airtight container and store in the refrigerator until ready to eat, up to 1 week.

SERVES 12	
Per Serving:	
Calories	186
Fat	19g
Protein	3g
Sodium	84mg
Fiber	1g
Carbohydrates	7g
Net Carbs	4g
Sugar	1g

Vanilla Ice Cream Fat Bomb Smoothie

If you're missing ice cream, make this smoothie. You can turn this into a coffee-flavored fat bomb smoothie by using frozen coffee cubes in place of the regular ice cubes.

12 ice cubes

3 cups unsweetened vanilla almond milk

2 tablespoons MCT oil powder

¼ cup coconut cream

2 teaspoons vanilla extract

2 tablespoons granulated erythritol

1 Combine all ingredients in a blender and blend until smooth.

2 Pour equal amounts into two cups and serve immediately.

Cinnamon Roll Fat Bomb Smoothie

This smoothie is easy to whip up with just a few staple keto ingredients. If you keep your pantry well stocked, you'll be able to make it when the need for an extra boost of fat strikes.

2 cups full-fat coconut milk

¼ cup keto-friendly vanilla protein powder

2 tablespoons MCT oil powder

1 teaspoon ground cinnamon

½ teaspoon vanilla extract

2 cups ice

1 Combine all ingredients in a blender and blend until smooth.

2 Pour into two cups and serve immediately.

CHAPTER 8

Keto Slow Cooker and Pressure Cooker Meals

Barbecue Pulled Pork

SERVES 12	
Per Serving:	
Calories	311
Fat	19g
Protein	31g
Sodium	1,050mg
Fiber	0g
Carbohydrates	0g
Net Carbs	0g
Sugar	0g

WHAT IS SAZÓN?

Sazón is the Spanish word for "seasoning." Most grocery stores sell a premade Sazón seasoning, but if you're having trouble finding one or you want to use up what's in your spice cabinet, you can make your own at home. Combine 1 tablespoon ground coriander, 1 tablespoon ground cumin, 1 tablespoon turmeric, 1 tablespoon garlic powder, 1 tablespoon sea salt, 2 teaspoons dried oregano, and 1 teaspoon ground black pepper. Use what you need and store the rest in an airtight container in your spice cabinet for up to 6 months.

You never have to miss barbecue with this keto-friendly recipe. Pair this Barbecue Pulled Pork with guacamole and Fresh Broccoli Slaw (see recipe in Chapter 5) to make it a satisfying, balanced keto meal.

1 (4-pound) pork loin
3 tablespoons Sazón seasoning
½ cup beef bone broth
¾ cup keto-approved barbecue sauce

1 Pat pork dry with a paper towel and place on a cutting board. Sprinkle Sazón seasoning all over pork, covering as much as possible.

2 Pour beef broth into slow cooker and place seasoned pork on top. Cook on low for 8 hours.

3 Remove pork from slow cooker and shred with two forks. Return shredded pork to slow cooker.

4 Pour barbecue sauce on top of shredded pork and stir to mix. Cook on low for another 30 minutes.

5 Remove from heat and serve.

Greek Lemon Chicken

This Greek Lemon Chicken comes together simply and quickly with ingredients you probably already have on hand.

¼ cup fresh lemon juice

1½ teaspoons lemon zest

1 tablespoon Greek seasoning

½ teaspoon oregano

½ teaspoon sea salt

½ teaspoon ground black pepper

2 tablespoons olive oil

1 pound boneless, skinless chicken tenders

SERVES 4	
Per Serving:	
Calories	372
Fat	23g
Protein	22g
Sodium	1,130mg
Fiber	2g
Carbohydrates	21g
Net Carbs	19g
Sugar	1g

1 Place all ingredients except chicken in a small bowl and whisk until combined. Place chicken in slow cooker and pour lemon juice mixture on top. Cook on low for 5 hours.

2 Remove chicken from slow cooker and shred with two forks. Return shredded chicken to slow cooker and stir to coat with sauce. Cook on low for another 30 minutes. Serve hot.

Beef Curry

You need only five simple ingredients to whip up this delicious Beef Curry. Serve it on top of Curried Cauliflower or with some Simmered Collard Greens (see recipes in Chapter 5) for a complete keto meal.

2 tablespoons curry powder

2 pounds beef stew meat

1 cup coconut cream

2 tablespoons tomato paste

1 medium yellow onion, peeled and roughly chopped

SERVES 6	
Per Serving:	
Calories	371
Fat	24g
Protein	32g
Sodium	148mg
Fiber	2g
Carbohydrates	6g
Net Carbs	4g
Sugar	3g

1 Sprinkle curry powder over stew meat, tossing to coat as much as possible.

2 Add coconut cream and tomato paste to slow cooker and whisk to combine. Place seasoned stew meat in slow cooker and sprinkle onions on top.

3 Cook on low for 8 hours. Serve hot.

Spicy Thai Pork Roast

FRESH VERSUS DRIED HERBS AND SPICES

You can usually substitute dried herbs for fresh, but you have to adjust the amounts. Dried versions are concentrated and, because of this, a lot more potent. When a recipe calls for fresh spices or herbs, you want to use about one-third of the amount if you're using dried. For example, if a recipe calls for 1 tablespoon fresh chives, you would use 1 teaspoon dried chives in its place.

This pork roast isn't too spicy, but it does have a nice kick that comes from the ginger. If you don't have fresh ginger, you can substitute it with dried ginger, but reduce the amount by amount one-third.

2 teaspoons sea salt

1 teaspoon granulated garlic

¾ teaspoon granulated onion

1 teaspoon white pepper

½ teaspoon ground ginger

1 (2-pound) pork loin

2 tablespoons avocado oil

1 tablespoon minced garlic

1 tablespoon minced ginger

¼ cup no-sugar-added creamy almond butter

¼ cup tomato sauce

3 tablespoons coconut aminos

¼ cup granulated erythritol

1 tablespoon Thai chili garlic paste

¼ cup chicken bone broth

1 Combine spices in a small bowl. Spread spice mixture all over pork loin, covering as much as possible.

2 Heat avocado oil in a medium cast iron skillet over medium-high heat. Cook pork on each side for 2 to 3 minutes or until browned. Transfer pork to a slow cooker.

3 Combine remaining ingredients in a food processor. Process until smooth, about 2 minutes.

4 Pour sauce over pork. Cook on low for 3 hours or until internal temperature of pork reaches 145°F.

5 Remove pork from slow cooker and let rest for 10 minutes. Slice pork into medallions and pour sauce from slow cooker on top before serving.

Shrimp Scampi

You can turn this Shrimp Scampi into a seafood scampi by using a combination of shrimp and scallops, instead of shrimp alone. Use pinot grigio, sauvignon blanc, or chardonnay, which have only around 1 to 2 grams of carbs per ¼ cup, and pair it with your favorite keto-friendly pasta substitute, like spaghetti squash or zucchini noodles.

½ cup chicken bone broth

¼ cup keto-friendly dry white wine

¼ cup grass-fed butter

1 tablespoon lemon juice

1½ tablespoons minced garlic

½ teaspoon sea salt

¼ teaspoon ground black pepper

½ teaspoon crushed red pepper

1 pound raw large shrimp, peeled and deveined

½ cup grated Parmesan cheese

1 tablespoon chopped fresh parsley

1 Combine broth, wine, butter, lemon juice, garlic, salt, black pepper, and red pepper in a 2-quart slow cooker. Add shrimp, toss to coat, and cover.

2 Cook on low for 2 hours.

3 Transfer shrimp and sauce to a plate. Sprinkle Parmesan cheese and fresh parsley on top.

SERVES 4	
Per Serving:	
Calories	294
Fat	18g
Protein	28g
Sodium	1,376mg
Fiber	0g
Carbohydrates	2g
Net Carbs	2g
Sugar	0g

THE SELENIUM IN SHRIMP

Shrimp is highly nutritious, offering more than twenty different vitamins and minerals per serving, but the content of one specific mineral—selenium—is most notable. One 4-ounce serving of shrimp provides all of the selenium you need for the entire day. Selenium helps reduce inflammation, promotes heart health, and keeps your thyroid running as it should. Research shows that many people with thyroid diseases are actually deficient in selenium.

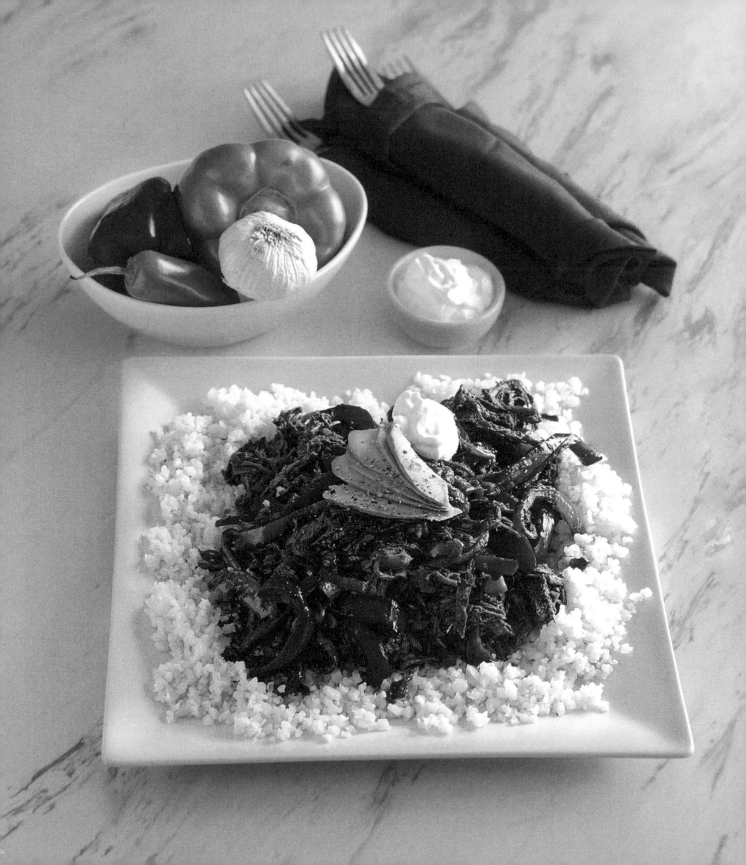

Steak Fajitas

These Steak Fajitas are so flavorful that you won't even miss the tortillas! Try serving them over a bed of cauliflower rice, topped with sliced avocado, and with a dollop of sour cream.

2 teaspoons cumin

½ teaspoon smoked paprika

2 pounds skirt steak

¼ cup beef bone broth

1 small yellow onion, peeled and sliced into strips

1 medium red bell pepper, seeded and sliced into strips

1 medium green bell pepper, seeded and sliced into strips

2 medium jalapeños, seeded and diced

1 tablespoon apple cider vinegar

¼ cup no-sugar-added ketchup

1½ teaspoons minced garlic

½ teaspoon sea salt

¼ teaspoon ground black pepper

SERVES 6	
Per Serving:	
Calories	291
Fat	16g
Protein	33g
Sodium	412mg
Fiber	1g
Carbohydrates	5g
Net Carbs	4g
Sugar	2g

1 Combine cumin and paprika in a small bowl and sprinkle over steak, coating as much as possible.

2 Pour broth in slow cooker and place steak on top. Add onions and peppers.

3 Whisk remaining ingredients together in a small bowl. Pour on top of onions and peppers and cover.

4 Cook for 3 hours on low, stir, replace cover, and cook for an additional 3 hours on low.

5 Remove steak from slow cooker and shred with two forks. Return to slow cooker and stir. Serve hot.

Lemon Pepper Pork Tenderloin

SERVES 6

Per Serving:

Calories	227
Fat	10g
Protein	31g
Sodium	422mg
Fiber	0g
Carbohydrates	1g
Net Carbs	1g
Sugar	0g

THE THICKENING POWER OF ARROWROOT

Arrowroot starch, also called *arrowroot powder* or *arrowroot flour*, is naturally gluten-free, grain-free, vegan, and paleo-approved. It comes from the root of a tropical plant called *Maranta arundinacea*. A common use is as a thickener. Unlike cornstarch, arrowroot starch has no taste. It also has more thickening power than cornstarch, so when you replace cornstarch with arrowroot starch, you want to start with one-third to one-half the amount of cornstarch the recipe calls for.

The arrowroot starch used in this recipe thickens the juice up a little bit so you can use it as a sauce. If you don't have arrowroot starch, or you don't have room in your carbohydrate allotment for it, you can simply leave it out.

1 teaspoon minced garlic

1 (2-pound) pork tenderloin

1 teaspoon sea salt

1 teaspoon ground black pepper

2 tablespoons fresh lemon juice

2 tablespoons olive oil

1 teaspoon arrowroot starch

2 teaspoons water

1 Rub garlic all over pork tenderloin. Combine salt and pepper in a small bowl. Sprinkle over pork tenderloin, covering as much as possible.

2 Add seasoned pork to slow cooker and pour lemon juice and olive oil on top.

3 Cover and cook on low for 4 hours or until internal temperature of pork reaches 145°F. Remove pork from slow cooker and allow to rest for 10 minutes.

4 Turn slow cooker to high. Whisk together arrowroot starch and water. Whisk arrowroot mixture into sauce in the slow cooker and continue whisking for 5 minutes or until sauce starts to thicken.

5 Slice pork into medallions and pour sauce on top. Serve hot.

Loaded Smashed Cauliflower

This dish has all the richness of mashed potatoes but without any of the carbs—the best of both worlds!

1 large head cauliflower, cut into florets

2 teaspoons minced garlic

1 teaspoon dried rosemary

1 teaspoon sea salt

½ teaspoon ground black pepper

1 cup chicken bone broth

½ cup sour cream

½ cup shredded Cheddar cheese

2 scallions, chopped, green part only

SERVES 6	
Per Serving:	
Calories	110
Fat	7g
Protein	6g
Sodium	487mg
Fiber	2g
Carbohydrates	6g
Net Carbs	4g
Sugar	2g

1 Place cauliflower in slow cooker. Add garlic, rosemary, salt, pepper, and broth. Cook on low for 5 hours or until soft.

2 Drain excess liquid from slow cooker and add remaining ingredients, except scallions. Use an immersion blender to purée. Sprinkle scallions on top and serve hot.

Jamaican Jerk Pot Roast

Jamaican jerk seasoning is known for one major thing—spice! If you want to dial it down, reduce the amount of seasoning.

1 tablespoon olive oil

2 teaspoons minced garlic

1 (2-pound) pork shoulder

2 tablespoons Jamaican jerk seasoning

½ cup beef bone broth

SERVES 6	
Per Serving:	
Calories	330
Fat	22g
Protein	29g
Sodium	152mg
Fiber	0g
Carbohydrates	0g
Net Carbs	0g
Sugar	0g

1 Combine oil and garlic in a small bowl. Rub mixture all over pork shoulder. Sprinkle jerk seasoning over pork shoulder.

2 Add beef broth to slow cooker and place seasoned pork shoulder on top.

3 Cook on low for 6 hours. Remove pork from slow cooker, shred with two forks, and return to slow cooker. Mix to incorporate juices. Serve warm.

Cheesy Bacon Ranch Chicken

SERVES 6

Per Serving:

Calories	554
Fat	31g
Protein	48g
Sodium	940mg
Fiber	1g
Carbohydrates	6g
Net Carbs	5g
Sugar	1g

Cheese, bacon, and ranch—some of the best flavors to mix. This recipe combines all three together for a hearty meal that's easy to throw together.

1 tablespoon dried parsley

1 teaspoon dried dill

1 teaspoon granulated garlic

1 teaspoon granulated onion

¾ teaspoon sea salt

½ teaspoon ground black pepper

1 cup sour cream

2 pounds boneless, skinless chicken breasts

½ cup Tessemae's Organic Creamy Ranch Dressing

1 cup shredded Cheddar cheese

1 cup shredded Colby jack cheese

6 slices no-sugar-added bacon, cooked and chopped

1 Combine spices and sour cream in a small bowl and mix well. Spread sour cream mixture over chicken breasts and place in slow cooker.

2 Cook on low for 6 hours.

3 Shred chicken with two forks and stir in remaining ingredients. Cook for an additional 10 minutes. Serve hot.

Zucchini and Sausage Soup

This spicy Zucchini and Sausage Soup is loaded with low-carb vegetables to help boost your micronutrient intake. Plus, it's an excellent way to use up all that zucchini from your garden.

1½ pounds no-sugar-added hot Italian sausage

1½ cups chopped celery

2 pounds zucchini, julienned

2 (28-ounce) cans petite-diced tomatoes, drained

1 large green bell pepper, seeded and sliced

1 large red bell pepper, seeded and sliced

1 cup chopped peeled yellow onion

2 teaspoons sea salt

1 teaspoon Italian seasoning

1 teaspoon dried oregano

1 teaspoon dried basil

½ teaspoon dried thyme

½ teaspoon granulated garlic

SERVES 6	
Per Serving:	
Calories	324
Fat	18g
Protein	16g
Sodium	1,813mg
Fiber	7g
Carbohydrates	23g
Net Carbs	16g
Sugar	11g

1 Heat a medium skillet over medium-high heat. Crumble sausage into pan and cook until no longer pink, about 7 minutes. Add celery and continue cooking until celery softens, about 7 more minutes.

2 Transfer cooked sausage mixture to slow cooker and add remaining ingredients to slow cooker and stir to combine.

3 Cook on low for 5 hours. Serve hot.

Ropa Vieja

Ropa vieja is one of the national dishes of Cuba. Traditionally, it's served with white rice, but you can serve it with Cilantro Lime Cauliflower Rice (see recipe in Chapter 5) for a low-carb version that still has an authentic Cuban feel.

2 tablespoons avocado oil

1 (2-pound) beef chuck roast

1 (28-ounce) can fire-roasted diced tomatoes, drained

1 cup beef bone broth

2 yellow onions, peeled and sliced

1 large red bell pepper, seeded and sliced

1 large green bell pepper, seeded and sliced

1 large yellow bell pepper, seeded and sliced

1 small jalapeño, seeded and diced

1 (6-ounce) can tomato paste

2 tablespoons minced garlic

1 tablespoon olive oil

1 tablespoon red wine vinegar

1 teaspoon ground cumin

1 teaspoon sea salt

½ teaspoon white pepper

⅛ teaspoon cayenne pepper

¼ cup chopped fresh cilantro

1   Heat avocado oil in a large skillet over medium-high heat. Brown roast by cooking for 3 minutes on each side. Transfer roast to slow cooker.

2   Add tomatoes to slow cooker. Pour broth over roast and add onions, bell peppers, and jalapeño. Mix remaining ingredients, except cilantro, in a small bowl, and pour into slow cooker.

3   Cook on low for 8 hours or until roast is tender.

4   Remove roast from slow cooker and shred with two forks. Return beef to slow cooker and stir to mix with juices.

5   Cook for an additional 30 minutes. Remove from heat, garnish with cilantro, and serve hot.

Pernil Pork

Pernil *is the name for a slow-roasted, marinated pork leg or pork shoulder. It's commonly served during Christmas in Puerto Rico with a side of rice, or Arroz con Gandules.*

2 teaspoons minced garlic

1 large yellow onion, peeled and roughly chopped

1 teaspoon dried oregano

1 teaspoon granulated garlic

1 tablespoon ground cumin

2 teaspoons chili powder

1½ teaspoons sea salt

1½ teaspoons ground black pepper

¼ cup olive oil

1 tablespoon apple cider vinegar

1 (2-pound) boneless pork loin

SERVES 6	
Per Serving:	
Calories	410
Fat	29g
Protein	33g
Sodium	668mg
Fiber	1g
Carbohydrates	4g
Net Carbs	3g
Sugar	1g

1 Combine minced garlic, onion, oregano, granulated garlic, cumin, chili powder, salt, and pepper in a blender with olive oil and vinegar. Blend until smooth.

2 Rub mixture over pork loin and transfer to a slow cooker. Cook on low for 8 hours.

3 Remove pork from slow cooker and shred with two forks. Return to slow cooker and mix to combine with juices. Cook for an additional 30 minutes.

4 Remove from slow cooker and serve hot.

Spicy Salsa Chicken

SERVES 6

Per Serving:

Calories	153
Fat	2g
Protein	27g
Sodium	573mg
Fiber	2g
Carbohydrates	6g
Net Carbs	4g
Sugar	3g

A METABOLISM BOOST WITH CAPSAICIN

Research shows that capsaicin, the compound in chili peppers that makes them spicy, may help boost your metabolism, curb your appetite, and reduce the amount of fat tissue you have. The process it triggers is thermogenesis, and it works like this: When you eat spicy things, your core temperature rises (which is why you may sweat a little). In order to raise your core temperature, your body has to burn calories. Those calories generally come from your fat tissue.

If you want to up the fat content of this recipe a little bit, you can use chicken thighs in place of chicken breasts. Serve with Mexican-style cauliflower rice, which is cooked with diced tomatoes and cumin, and a dollop of good-quality sour cream.

2 teaspoons ground cumin

2 teaspoons chili powder

½ teaspoon paprika

½ teaspoon sea salt

¼ teaspoon ground black pepper

6 (4-ounce) boneless, skinless chicken breasts

1 (8-ounce) jar no-sugar-added hot salsa

½ cup tomato sauce

2 teaspoons minced garlic

1 small red onion, peeled and diced

1 Combine cumin, chili powder, paprika, salt, and pepper in a small bowl. Sprinkle over chicken, coating as much as possible.

2 Place chicken breasts in slow cooker. Pour salsa and tomato sauce on top. Add garlic and onion and cover.

3 Cook on low for 4 hours or until chicken is tender. Shred chicken with two forks and stir to combine.

4 Serve hot.

Spinach and Bacon Egg Bites

This recipe requires a silicone egg bite mold that fits into the pot of your pressure cooker. You can find this mold online or at many home supply stores.

4 large eggs

¾ cup grated Parmesan cheese

¼ cup full-fat coconut milk

¼ teaspoon sea salt

½ teaspoon ground black pepper

¼ cup packed chopped spinach

4 slices no-sugar-added bacon, cooked and chopped

SERVES 2	
Per Serving:	
Calories	459
Fat	35g
Protein	37g
Sodium	1,440mg
Fiber	0g
Carbohydrates	2g
Net Carbs	2g
Sugar	0g

1 Combine eggs, Parmesan cheese, coconut milk, salt, and pepper in a medium bowl and whisk until incorporated.

2 Sprinkle equal amounts of chopped spinach and bacon into each well of a silicone egg mold. Pour egg mixture on top of spinach and bacon, filling each well 80 percent of the way. Cover tightly with foil.

3 Add 1½ cups of water to the inner pot of a pressure cooker and place a trivet inside. Place mold on top of trivet and seal pressure cooker lid.

4 Cook for 10 minutes on high pressure. Allow pressure to release naturally for an additional 10 minutes. Manually release any remaining pressure.

5 Carefully remove egg mold from pressure cooker and remove egg bites from mold. Serve hot or cold.

Shrimp and Chicken Jambalaya

SERVES 6	
Per Serving:	
Calories	366
Fat	15g
Protein	41g
Sodium	1,546mg
Fiber	2g
Carbohydrates	12g
Net Carbs	10g
Sugar	5g

Traditional jambalaya, which comes from Louisiana, combines meat, sausage, and vegetables mixed with rice. This low-carb version uses those amazing flavors in a keto-friendly way!

2 tablespoons olive oil, divided

1 pound no-sugar-added andouille sausage, sliced into coins

1 large yellow onion, peeled and chopped

2 teaspoons minced garlic

1 pound boneless, skinless chicken breasts, cubed

1 medium green bell pepper, seeded and diced

3 medium stalks celery, diced

1 (28-ounce) can petite-diced tomatoes, drained

1 pound raw medium shrimp, peeled and deveined

1 teaspoon seasoned salt

½ teaspoon ground black pepper

¼ teaspoon cayenne pepper

1 Turn on the sauté function of your pressure cooker. Add 1 tablespoon olive oil to the pot and allow to heat. Add sausage and cook until browned, about 5 minutes. Remove sausage from the pot with a slotted spoon and set aside.

2 Add onion and garlic to pot and cook until softened, about 3 minutes. Add chicken, bell pepper, and celery and cook for 5 minutes or until chicken starts to brown. Add remaining 1 tablespoon olive oil, then the rest of the ingredients and browned sausage and stir.

3 Secure the lid of the pressure cooker and cook on high for 7 minutes.

4 Release pressure manually. Serve hot.

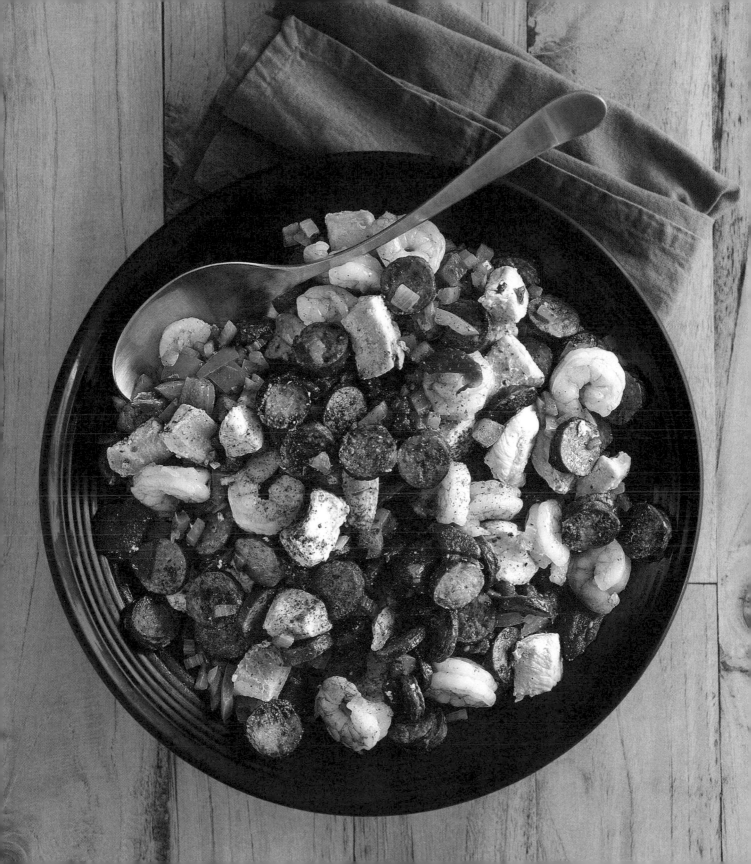

Lemon Garlic Chicken

SERVES 6

Per Serving:

Calories	206
Fat	9g
Protein	27g
Sodium	337mg
Fiber	1g
Carbohydrates	4g
Net Carbs	3g
Sugar	1g

WHAT'S NATURAL PRESSURE RELEASE?

When a pressure cooker recipe calls for natural release, it means that when the meal is done cooking, you should let the pressure release on its own, rather than turning the valve to release the pressure yourself. On the other hand, manual pressure release is when you open the pressure valve to release all the steam instead of letting it slowly seep out on its own. Allowing the pressure to release naturally typically lets the food cook longer.

This dish doesn't require sophisticated ingredients, but it tastes like it came from a fancy restaurant. Serve it with Spicy Parmesan Broccoli Rabe (see recipe in Chapter 5) for a real treat.

½ teaspoon sea salt

½ teaspoon ground black pepper

¼ teaspoon paprika

1 teaspoon granulated garlic

¼ teaspoon onion salt

1½ pounds boneless, skinless chicken breasts, cubed

1 tablespoon olive oil

2 tablespoons grass-fed butter

1 small yellow onion, peeled and roughly chopped

1½ teaspoons minced garlic

¼ cup chicken bone broth

1 teaspoon dried oregano

1 teaspoon dried basil

2 tablespoons lemon juice

1 teaspoon lemon zest

2 tablespoons coconut cream

2 tablespoons water

2 teaspoons arrowroot powder

1 Combine salt, pepper, paprika, granulated garlic, and onion salt in a medium bowl. Add chicken to bowl and toss to coat.

2 Turn pressure cooker to sauté function and heat olive oil. Add chicken and cook until browned, about 5 minutes. Remove chicken from pot and set aside.

3 Add butter, onion, and minced garlic to pot and cook for 2 minutes, stirring and scraping the bottom of the pot to remove browned bits from the bottom. Add chicken broth, oregano, basil, lemon juice, and lemon zest and stir to combine.

4 Return chicken to pot and secure lid. Cook on high pressure for 7 minutes. Allow pressure to release naturally for 3 minutes and then release any remaining pressure manually. Remove lid. Remove chicken from pot.

5 Stir in coconut cream. Whisk water and arrowroot powder together in a small bowl and stir into sauce. Continue stirring for 3 minutes or until thickened. Pour sauce over chicken and serve hot.

Pesto Chicken

When you use bone-in chicken thighs, the flavor that's inside of the marrow in the bone seeps out into the meat, giving it a deeper, richer flavor. Not only that, but bone-in chicken is usually more wallet-friendly than boneless chicken since it requires less processing.

1 teaspoon sea salt

½ teaspoon ground black pepper

6 (4-ounce) bone-in chicken thighs, skins removed

1 tablespoon olive oil

1½ cups chicken bone broth

8 ounces cream cheese

2 cups chopped trimmed asparagus

½ cup keto-friendly basil pesto

½ teaspoon granulated garlic

½ teaspoon granulated onion

1 Sprinkle salt and pepper on chicken thighs and set aside.

2 Turn on the sauté function of your pressure cooker and add olive oil to the pot. When the olive oil is hot, add chicken and cook until chicken starts to brown, about 5 minutes.

3 Add chicken broth and secure lid. Cook on the poultry setting for 30 minutes. Release pressure manually.

4 Open the lid and add remaining ingredients. Stir to combine.

5 Secure lid and cook on high for an additional 3 minutes. Release pressure manually.

6 Remove the lid and allow chicken to cool slightly. Serve hot.

SERVES 6	
Per Serving:	
Calories	418
Fat	32g
Protein	26g
Sodium	805mg
Fiber	2g
Carbohydrates	7g
Net Carbs	5g
Sugar	2g

TROUBLESHOOTING YOUR PRESSURE COOKER

One of the most common error messages people get when using a pressure cooker is the "burn" or "scorch" error. Typically, that means one of two things. Something's either stuck to the bottom of the pot or there isn't enough liquid in it. You can rectify this error message by manually releasing all the pressure, opening your pressure cooker and scraping off any browned bits stuck to the pot and adding a little more liquid, such as broth, juices from a tomato can, water, or coconut milk.

Cream of Asparagus Soup

If you eat dairy, you can replace the coconut cream in this Cream of Asparagus Soup with some grass-fed half-and-half or heavy cream.

8 slices no-sugar-added bacon, chopped

1 small yellow onion, peeled and diced

2 teaspoons minced garlic

3 pounds asparagus, trimmed and cut into 1-inch pieces

4 cups chicken bone broth

2 teaspoons sea salt

1 teaspoon ground black pepper

1½ cups coconut cream

1 Turn on sauté function of pressure cooker. Add bacon and cook until bacon starts to brown, about 3 minutes. Add onion and garlic and cook for another 3 minutes. Add asparagus and continue cooking until it starts to soften, about 3 minutes.

2 Pour chicken broth into pot and stir in salt and pepper. Bring to a boil and turn off pressure cooker.

3 Secure the lid and cook on high for 5 minutes. Allow pressure to release naturally and carefully remove lid.

4 Use an immersion blender to purée mixture until smooth. Stir in coconut cream. Serve hot.

Salmon Piccata

If you don't have herbes de Provence seasoning, you can season the sauce with rosemary, thyme, basil, marjoram, oregano, tarragon, parsley, or any combination of dried or fresh herbs that you like.

1 teaspoon sea salt

½ teaspoon ground black pepper

2 (4-ounce) salmon fillets

½ cup water

2 tablespoons grass-fed butter

1 tablespoon minced garlic

1 cup chicken bone broth

2 teaspoons arrowroot powder

¼ cup coconut cream

2 tablespoons lemon juice

1 teaspoon herbes de Provence seasoning

¼ teaspoon dried minced onion

2 tablespoons capers

SERVES 2	
Per Serving:	
Calories	401
Fat	29g
Protein	25g
Sodium	1,444mg
Fiber	1g
Carbohydrates	6g
Net Carbs	5g
Sugar	1g

1 Sprinkle salt and pepper on salmon and set salmon on top of a trivet in your pressure cooker. Add water to the pot.

2 Secure the lid and cook on the steam setting for 15 minutes.

3 While salmon is cooking, add butter and garlic to a medium skillet over medium heat. Cook for 4 minutes or until garlic starts to turn golden brown. Add chicken broth, arrowroot powder, coconut cream, lemon juice, herb seasoning, onion, and capers to the skillet. Stir to combine.

4 Reduce heat to low and continue cooking until sauce thickens, about 5 minutes, stirring frequently.

5 When salmon is done cooking, allow pressure to release naturally. Remove lid and transfer salmon fillets to a plate. Spoon sauce on top. Serve hot.

Creamy Sausage and Cabbage Soup

Per Serving:

Calories	591
Fat	49g
Protein	24g
Sodium	1,118mg
Fiber	2g
Carbohydrates	10g
Net Carbs	8g
Sugar	4g

THE CRUCIFEROUS CABBAGE

Cabbage has more to offer than just a low carbohydrate count. That same serving also provides about half of the amount of vitamin C you need for the entire day and about 75 percent of the amount of vitamin K. According to research published in *Nutrition and Cancer,* eating cabbage can also reduce your risk of certain cancers, like stomach and esophageal cancer.

Cabbage is a staple on a keto diet, and for good reason. One cup of chopped raw cabbage contains only 5 grams of carbohydrates, 2.2 grams of which come from fiber.

3 tablespoons grass-fed butter

1 large yellow onion, peeled and chopped

1 teaspoon minced garlic

1½ pounds no-sugar-added sage pork sausage

1½ cups chicken bone broth

3 cups chopped cabbage

½ teaspoon garlic salt

½ teaspoon ground black pepper

⅛ teaspoon cayenne pepper

1½ cups full-fat coconut milk

1 tablespoon arrowroot powder

1 Turn on the sauté function of your pressure cooker. Add butter. Once butter is hot, add onion and garlic and cook for 4 minutes. Add sausage and cook until no longer pink, about 7 minutes.

2 Add chicken broth, cabbage, garlic salt, black pepper, and cayenne pepper and stir to combine. Secure the lid and cook on high pressure for 9 minutes. Release pressure manually.

3 Remove lid carefully and turn sauté function back on. Stir in coconut milk and arrowroot powder and cook for 5 minutes or until soup thickens slightly. Serve hot.

Sweet and Spicy Baby Back Ribs

The days of having to cook ribs for hours are over. With the help of a pressure cooker, you can have these Sweet and Spicy Baby Back Ribs on the table in less than 45 minutes. Serve them with some Fresh Broccoli Slaw (see recipe in Chapter 5) for an authentic barbecue pairing.

¼ cup brown granulated erythritol

2 tablespoons chili powder

2 teaspoons dried parsley

1½ teaspoons sea salt

1½ teaspoons granulated garlic

1½ teaspoons granulated onion

1½ teaspoons ground black pepper

1 teaspoon ground cumin

1 teaspoon smoked paprika

1½ pounds baby back ribs

¾ cup water

¼ cup apple cider vinegar

1 (12-ounce) bottle keto-friendly barbecue sauce

SERVES 6	
Per Serving:	
Calories	290
Fat	20g
Protein	17g
Sodium	1,006mg
Fiber	2g
Carbohydrates	12g
Net Carbs	2g
Sugar	0g

1 Combine erythritol, chili powder, parsley, salt, garlic, onion, pepper, cumin, and paprika in a small bowl. Rub spice mixture all over ribs, coating as much as possible.

2 Place trivet inside pot of pressure cooker and pour water and apple cider vinegar in the bottom of the pot. Place ribs on trivet and secure lid.

3 Cook on high pressure for 22 minutes and then release pressure manually. Remove lid carefully and transfer ribs to a baking sheet lined with aluminum foil.

4 Turn on oven's broiler. Pour barbecue sauce on top of ribs and broil until sauce is bubbly and hot, about 4 minutes. Serve warm.

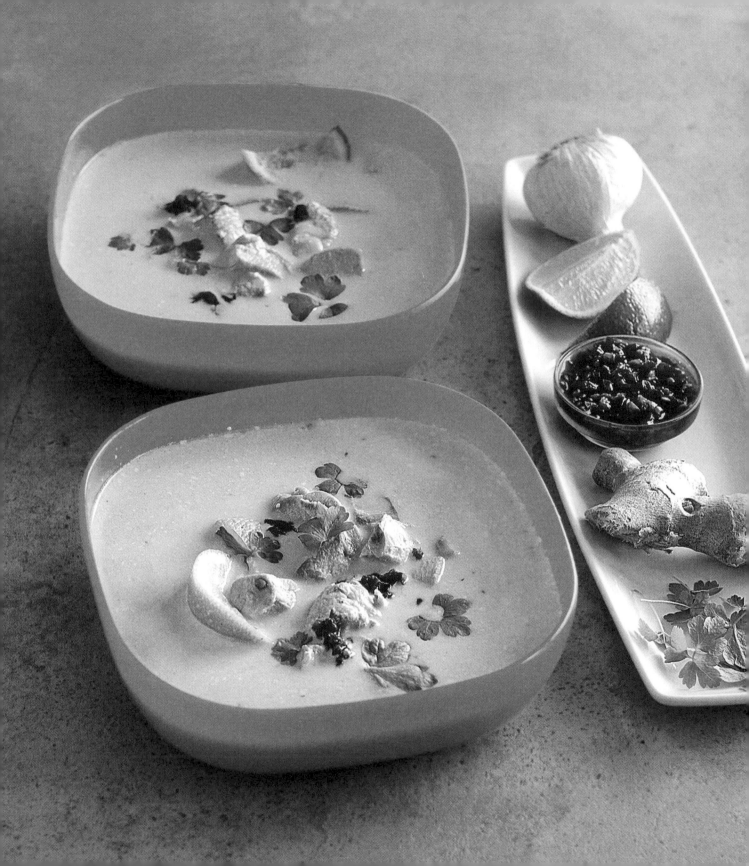

Tom Kha Gai

Tom Kha Gai is a coconut chicken soup that's one of the most popular dishes in Thailand. This version combines ginger and lime, which give you a kick, with a nice creaminess from the coconut milk.

1½ pounds boneless, skinless chicken breasts, cubed

2½ cups chicken bone broth

½ cup keto-friendly white wine

2 (14-ounce) cans coconut cream

2 tablespoons Thai garlic chili paste

1 tablespoon coconut aminos

2 teaspoons lime juice

1 teaspoon sea salt

1 teaspoon ground ginger

2 tablespoons chopped fresh cilantro

SERVES 6	
Per Serving:	
Calories	624
Fat	23g
Protein	31g
Sodium	731mg
Fiber	0g
Carbohydrates	2g
Net Carbs	2g
Sugar	1g

1 Combine all ingredients, except cilantro, in the pot of a pressure cooker. Secure the lid and cook on the soup function for 30 minutes. Allow pressure to release naturally for 5 minutes, then release any remaining pressure manually.

2 Remove lid and stir in fresh cilantro. Serve hot.

Whole Lemon Chicken

SERVES 6	
Per Serving:	
Calories	289
Fat	18g
Protein	29g
Sodium	647mg
Fiber	0g
Carbohydrates	1g
Net Carbs	1g
Sugar	0g

When you're seasoning this chicken, lift the skin up a little and season in between the skin and the meat. This allows the flavor to penetrate the chicken a little more. You can even add a few extra teaspoons of butter in between the skin and the meat for extra fat and flavor.

2 lemons, sliced

1 (3-pound) whole chicken

2 tablespoons olive oil

1½ teaspoons sea salt

1½ teaspoons granulated garlic

1 teaspoon paprika

½ teaspoon lemon pepper

¼ teaspoon ground black pepper

1 cup chicken bone broth

1 Insert lemon slices into chicken cavity and set aside. Combine olive oil, salt, garlic, paprika, lemon pepper, and black pepper in a small bowl. Rub mixture all over the chicken, coating as much as possible.

2 Turn pressure cooker on to sauté function. When pot is hot, place chicken, breast side down, in the pot and cook until browned, about 4 minutes. Flip chicken over and cook for 4 more minutes, browning other side. Remove chicken from pot and set aside.

3 Pour chicken broth into pot and use a wooden spoon to scrape up any browned bits in the bottom of the pot. Place trivet in pot and put chicken on top, breast side down.

4 Secure the lid and cook on high pressure for 21 minutes. Allow pressure to release naturally.

5 Remove lid carefully and allow chicken to cool slightly. Remove from pressure cooker and serve hot.

Pork Chops and Gravy

These Pork Chops and Gravy call for cream of mushroom soup, but make sure not to use the processed stuff in a can. Homemade cream of mushroom soup is easy to make, tastes way better, and contains only healthy, keto-friendly ingredients.

2 tablespoons olive oil

1 teaspoon sea salt

½ teaspoon ground black pepper

6 bone-in pork chops

1 teaspoon minced garlic

½ cup chopped baby bella mushrooms

¼ cup keto-friendly dry white wine

¾ cup Keto-Friendly Cream of Mushroom Soup (see sidebar)

1¼ cups plus 2 tablespoons water, divided

1 tablespoon arrowroot powder

1 teaspoon coconut aminos

1 Turn pressure cooker on to sauté function and heat olive oil. Sprinkle salt and pepper on pork chops. Add pork chops to the pot in batches, cooking for 10 minutes, flipping each pork chop halfway through. Set pork chops aside.

2 Add garlic to pot and cook for 1 minute. Add mushrooms and cook until softened, about 5 minutes. Pour wine into pot and stir with a wooden spoon, scraping up any browned bits on the bottom of the pan. Cook for 5 minutes.

3 Stir in mushroom soup and 1¼ cups water and stir until smooth. Add pork chops and toss to coat. Secure lid.

4 Cook for 17 minutes on high pressure, then allow pressure to release naturally. Remove pork chops from the pot and set aside.

5 Turn pot back on to sauté function. Whisk together arrowroot powder and 2 tablespoons water in a small bowl and stir into sauce. Cook until thickened, about 5 minutes, stirring frequently. Stir in coconut aminos.

6 Pour sauce over pork chops and serve hot.

SERVES 6

Per Serving:

Calories	690
Fat	42g
Protein	66g
Sodium	957mg
Fiber	1g
Carbohydrates	6g
Net Carbs	5g
Sugar	2g

KETO-FRIENDLY SOUP

Canned cream of mushroom soup is full of wheat flour and starch. Make your own version by combining 1 tablespoon olive oil, ½ cup minced onion, 8 ounces sliced white mushrooms, 1½ teaspoons sea salt, ⅛ teaspoon garlic powder, ⅛ teaspoon ground black pepper, ½ cup chicken bone broth, 1 teaspoon chopped thyme, and ½ cup sour cream in a medium saucepan over medium-high heat. Cook until thickened, about 10 minutes.

Sloppy Joes

You can use brown erythritol or golden monk fruit sweetener for these Sloppy Joes. The brown sweeteners taste the most similar to brown sugar, which has added molasses and a richer taste than white sweeteners.

1 tablespoon olive oil

1 teaspoon minced garlic

1 small yellow onion, peeled and minced

1 medium red bell pepper, seeded and minced

1½ pounds 85/15 ground beef

1 teaspoon sea salt

½ teaspoon ground black pepper

¼ cup apple cider vinegar

¼ cup beef bone broth

2 tablespoons brown erythritol

1 teaspoon dry mustard powder

1 tablespoon coconut aminos

2 tablespoons tomato paste

1 tablespoon chili powder

¼ teaspoon crushed red pepper

1 (14.5-ounce) can petite-diced tomatoes, drained

1 Turn pressure cooker on to sauté function and add oil to pot. When oil is hot, add garlic, onion, and bell pepper. Cook until peppers start to soften, about 5 minutes. Add beef and cook until no longer pink, about 7 minutes. Season with salt and black pepper.

2 Stir in remaining ingredients and secure lid.

3 Cook for 5 minutes on high pressure. Allow pressure to release naturally for 10 minutes, then release any remaining pressure manually.

4 Allow to cool slightly and serve hot.

Bacon Cheddar Soup

White pepper is made by removing the outer layer from a black peppercorn before or after drying, leaving only the inner seed. White pepper has more of a kick than black pepper, but if you don't have it, you can use black pepper, which has a more complex flavor.

1 tablespoon olive oil

8 slices no-sugar-added bacon, diced

1 large yellow onion, peeled and diced

1½ teaspoons minced garlic

1 large head cauliflower, roughly chopped

2 teaspoons onion powder

1 teaspoon sea salt

½ teaspoon white pepper

1 teaspoon dry mustard powder

⅛ teaspoon cayenne pepper

4 cups chicken bone broth

2 cups shredded Cheddar cheese

1 cup heavy cream

SERVES 6	
Per Serving:	
Calories	433
Fat	34g
Protein	22g
Sodium	1,060mg
Fiber	2g
Carbohydrates	9g
Net Carbs	7g
Sugar	4g

1 Turn pressure cooker on to sauté function. Add olive oil.

2 When oil is hot, add bacon to pot and cook until bacon starts to brown, about 5 minutes. Add onion and garlic and cook for another 3 minutes.

3 Add cauliflower, onion powder, salt, white pepper, mustard powder, cayenne pepper, and chicken broth and stir to combine. Secure lid.

4 Cook on the soup setting for 15 minutes. Release pressure manually and carefully remove lid.

5 Stir in Cheddar cheese and cream. Serve hot.

Buffalo Chicken Meatballs

KEEPING YOUR HEART HEALTHY

Grass-fed butter is one of the richest dietary sources of vitamin K_2, a form of vitamin K that's been linked to lower risk of heart disease. In fact, researchers found that a diet high in vitamin K_2 can reduce your risk of dying from heart disease by as much as 57 percent, while reducing your risk of dying from other lifestyle diseases, like diabetes, by as much as 26 percent.

Enjoy these Buffalo Chicken Meatballs as a snack with a side of keto-friendly ranch or blue cheese dressing. You can also use them as an easy spicy protein source for your Mason jar salads.

1½ pounds ground chicken

¾ cup almond meal

1 teaspoon sea salt

¼ teaspoon dried parsley

1 teaspoon minced garlic

1 green onion, minced

6 tablespoons grass-fed butter, divided

6 tablespoons Frank's RedHot Original Cayenne Pepper Sauce

1 Combine chicken, almond meal, salt, parsley, garlic, and green onion in a medium bowl and mix with your hands until incorporated.

2 Wet hands and form mixture into 1-inch round meatballs.

3 Turn pressure cooker on to sauté function and add two tablespoons of butter. When butter is hot, add meatballs in batches, cooking for 2 minutes on each side or until browned.

4 Combine remaining butter and hot sauce in a small saucepan over medium heat. Stir until smooth.

5 Transfer all browned meatballs to pressure cooker and pour buffalo sauce on top.

6 Secure lid and cook on poultry setting for 17 minutes. Release pressure manually.

7 Carefully remove lid, allow meatballs to cool slightly, and serve hot.

CHAPTER 9

Keto Vegetarian and Vegan Meals

VE = Vegan VG = Vegetarian

Blackberry Yogurt Bowl

VE VG

SERVES 1

Per Serving:

Calories	511
Fat	35g
Protein	13g
Sodium	27mg
Fiber	10g
Carbohydrates	21g
Net Carbs	11g
Sugar	7g

This is a basic recipe that you can adapt to your own tastes by using any combination of your favorite keto-friendly yogurt options.

6 ounces plain full-fat coconut yogurt

¼ cup blackberries, divided

1 tablespoon hemp seeds

1 tablespoon sliced almonds

1 tablespoon flaked toasted coconut

1 tablespoon vegan stevia-sweetened chocolate chips

2 tablespoons no-sugar-added almond butter, melted

1 Combine yogurt and four blackberries in a food processor and process until smooth. Transfer mixture to a medium bowl.

2 Top with remaining blackberries, hemp seeds, almonds, coconut, and chocolate chips. Drizzle melted no-sugar-added almond butter on top. Serve immediately.

Cinnamon Roll Smoothie

VE VG

SERVES 1

Per Serving:

Calories	646
Fat	65g
Protein	8g
Sodium	56mg
Fiber	6g
Carbohydrates	10g
Net Carbs	4g
Sugar	4g

This delicious smoothie will curb your craving for the traditional sugar- and carb-loaded cinnamon roll. If you don't have fractionated coconut oil, you can melt a tablespoon of coconut oil, wait for it to cool slightly, and then add it to your smoothie. Try not to pour it into cold liquid or over the frozen avocado or it will just harden back up.

¾ cup full-fat coconut milk

¼ cup frozen avocado

½ teaspoon vanilla extract

¼ teaspoon ground cinnamon

1 tablespoon fractionated coconut oil

1 tablespoon hemp hearts

1 tablespoon vanilla MCT oil powder

1 Combine all ingredients in a blender and blend until smooth.

2 Serve immediately.

Blueberry Almond Overnight "Oats"

You may want to add more coconut milk right before eating to reach your desired consistency. Be mindful of the amount of blueberries you add. You can have a bit on your keto days, but don't overdo it.

⅔ cup full-fat coconut milk

½ cup hemp hearts

1 tablespoon chia seeds

2 teaspoons monk fruit-sweetened maple syrup

¼ teaspoon vanilla extract

⅛ teaspoon almond extract

⅛ teaspoon sea salt

2 tablespoons crushed almonds

1 tablespoon frozen wild blueberries

SERVES 2	
Per Serving:	
Calories	580
Fat	53g
Protein	18g
Sodium	187mg
Fiber	8g
Carbohydrates	13g
Net Carbs	1g
Sugar	3g

1 Combine all ingredients in a medium bowl and mix well.

2 Divide mixture in half and pour into two 16-ounce Mason jars. Cover and refrigerate overnight. Serve cold.

Spiced Chocolate Breakfast Milkshake

The cayenne pepper gives this milkshake a flavor that's reminiscent of Mexican hot chocolate. You can turn this into a hot drink by omitting the avocado and adding some granulated monk fruit sweetener to your tastes and combining them in a saucepan over low heat.

¾ cup full-fat coconut milk

¼ cup chopped frozen avocado

2 teaspoons unsweetened cocoa powder

½ teaspoon ground cinnamon

¼ teaspoon vanilla extract

1/16 teaspoon cayenne pepper

2 teaspoons chocolate MCT oil powder

SERVES 1	
Per Serving:	
Calories	566
Fat	55g
Protein	8g
Sodium	348mg
Fiber	11g
Carbohydrates	17g
Net Carbs	6g
Sugar	5g

1 Combine all ingredients in a blender and blend until smooth.

2 Serve immediately.

(VE) (VG)

Maple Brown Sugar "Oatmeal"

SERVES 1	
Per Serving:	
Calories	571
Fat	47g
Protein	15g
Sodium	206mg
Fiber	24g
Carbohydrates	46g
Net Carbs	1g
Sugar	4g

This is a base oatmeal-like recipe that you can tailor to your liking by adding any of your favorite keto-friendly toppings. Almonds, walnuts, and vegan stevia-sweetened chocolate chips all work nicely.

2½ tablespoons chia seeds

2½ tablespoons golden flax meal

2½ tablespoons shredded unsweetened coconut

¼ teaspoon ground cinnamon

1½ tablespoons golden monk fruit sweetener

⅔ cup full-fat coconut milk

2 tablespoons water

1½ tablespoons monk fruit–sweetened maple-flavored syrup

1 Combine chia seeds, flax meal, coconut, cinnamon, and golden monk fruit sweetener in a small bowl. Set aside.

2 Heat coconut milk and water in a small saucepan over medium-low heat for 3 minutes or until heated through. Stir in maple syrup.

3 Pour hot milk mixture over chia seed mixture and stir. Let sit for 5 minutes.

4 Stir and serve.

Peanut Butter Smoothie Bowl

This recipe is vegan as written. If you're vegetarian, you can replace the coconut yogurt with regular full-fat yogurt, which may be easier to find. If you're enjoying this Peanut Butter Smoothie Bowl on one of your high-carb days, you can add some frozen banana to the smoothie mixture before blending.

½ cup full-fat coconut milk

½ cup ice

¼ cup full-fat coconut yogurt

3 tablespoons no-sugar-added creamy peanut butter, divided

2 teaspoons chia seeds

½ teaspoon vanilla extract

1 tablespoon cacao nibs

1 tablespoon hemp hearts

1 tablespoon chopped peanuts

1 Combine coconut milk, ice, yogurt, 2 tablespoons peanut butter, chia seeds, and vanilla extract in a blender and blend until smooth. Transfer mixture to a small bowl.

2 Melt remaining peanut butter in a small saucepan over medium-low heat and drizzle on top of smoothie mixture. Top with cacao nibs, hemp hearts, and peanuts.

SERVES 1

Per Serving:

Calories	744
Fat	63g
Protein	22g
Sodium	64mg
Fiber	13g
Carbohydrates	23g
Net Carbs	10g
Sugar	8g

HEMP HEARTS

Hemp hearts are small, but mighty. A tablespoon contains 10 grams of protein and 12 grams of essential fatty acids (omega-3 and omega-6), which is more than a comparable serving of chia or flax. When blended into smoothies, hemp hearts add a subtle nutty taste. When combined with hot liquid, they take on a texture that's similar to that of oatmeal, making them a great low-carb alternative to the grain.

Vanilla Protein Pancakes

The type of protein powder you use in these pancakes will make a difference in the consistency. You can add a little more almond milk to thin it out or reduce the amount to make it thicker.

2 large eggs, separated

½ cup keto-friendly vegetarian vanilla protein powder

¼ teaspoon ground cinnamon

¼ teaspoon baking powder

¼ teaspoon sea salt

¼ teaspoon vanilla extract

2 tablespoons unsweetened vanilla almond milk

¼ cup frozen wild blueberries

2 tablespoons butter-flavored coconut oil

1 Place egg whites in a medium mixing bowl and beat with a hand-held mixer on high for 2 minutes or until soft peaks form. Set aside.

2 Put egg yolks in a medium bowl with remaining ingredients, except coconut oil, and whisk to combine.

3 Slowly fold egg whites into batter mixture, stirring just enough to incorporate.

4 Heat coconut oil in a medium skillet over medium heat. Use a ¼-cup measure to scoop mixture into hot pan. Cook for 1 minute on each side or until browned and cooked through.

5 Remove from heat and serve immediately.

SERVES 2

Per Serving:

Calories	444
Fat	21g
Protein	54g
Sodium	880mg
Fiber	2g
Carbohydrates	9g
Net Carbs	7g
Sugar	2g

CHOOSING A PROTEIN POWDER

You'll have to use extra care when choosing a protein powder for your keto lifestyle. Many protein powders contain added sugars to sweeten them and make them more palatable, but these sugars will throw your body out of ketosis with one scoop. 22 Days Nutrition and Vega are two companies that make natural, vegan, and keto-friendly protein powders. If you eat fish, you can choose a collagen protein that's sourced from marine bones instead of bovine (or beef) bones.

Breaded Zucchini Sticks

These easy-to-make sticks are favorites with kids and adults alike. If you want a sharper flavor, you can add a little grated Parmesan cheese to the breading mixture for a little extra fat and extra salty flavor.

⅓ cup paleo flour

½ teaspoon garlic powder

½ teaspoon onion salt

½ teaspoon dried parsley

¼ teaspoon paprika

¼ teaspoon sea salt

¼ teaspoon ground black pepper

2 medium zucchini, cut into 3" spears

3 large eggs, whisked

2 tablespoons butter-flavored coconut oil, melted

¼ cup Tessemae's Organic Habanero Ranch Dressing

1 Preheat air fryer to 400°F.

2 Combine paleo flour, garlic powder, onion salt, parsley, paprika, salt, and pepper in a medium bowl and mix until incorporated.

3 Dip zucchini spears in whisked egg and then toss in flour mixture to coat completely.

4 Arrange zucchini in basket of air fryer and drizzle melted coconut oil on top. Cook for 15 minutes or until zucchini is tender and breading is crispy. Serve warm with dressing on the side for dipping.

SERVES 2	
Per Serving:	
Calories	508
Fat	34g
Protein	15g
Sodium	1,041mg
Fiber	4g
Carbohydrates	17g
Net Carbs	13g
Sugar	5g

WHAT'S THE BUTTER FLAVOR?

Recently, a couple manufacturers (Nutiva and Thrive Market) have developed their own butter-flavored coconut oil. It gives the rich taste of butter, without any of the sweetness of coconut oil. The butter flavor is vegan and made from a combination of fermented plants, including sunflower, coconut, and mint. It's a great choice in savory dishes if you don't like the lingering taste of coconut.

Stuffed Pepper Omelets

SERVES 2

Per Serving:	
Calories	176
Fat	13g
Protein	12g
Sodium	391mg
Fiber	1g
Carbohydrates	4g
Net Carbs	3g
Sugar	2g

If you don't have an air fryer, you can cook these peppers in the oven instead. Line a baking sheet with parchment paper and cook for 45 minutes at 375°F or until eggs are set and peppers are softened.

½ cup whipped cream cheese, softened

½ cup shredded mozzarella cheese

¼ cup grated Parmesan cheese

½ teaspoon garlic powder

¼ teaspoon onion salt

¼ teaspoon dried parsley

⅛ teaspoon crushed red pepper

6 large eggs, whisked

¼ cup cooked broccoli florets

1 large orange bell pepper, sliced in half lengthwise and seeds removed

2 teaspoons Frank's RedHot Original Cayenne Pepper Sauce

1 Preheat air fryer to 350°F.

2 Place cream cheese in a medium mixing bowl and beat with a handheld mixer until light and fluffy, about 1 minute. Add mozzarella cheese, Parmesan cheese, garlic powder, onion salt, parsley, and red pepper to bowl with cream cheese and beat on low until just combined. Add eggs and broccoli and stir to combine.

3 Arrange peppers cut side up in the basket of your air fryer. Divide mixture in half and scoop equal parts into each half of pepper.

4 Cook in the air fryer for 30 minutes or until eggs are set.

5 Remove from basket, splash with hot sauce, and serve warm.

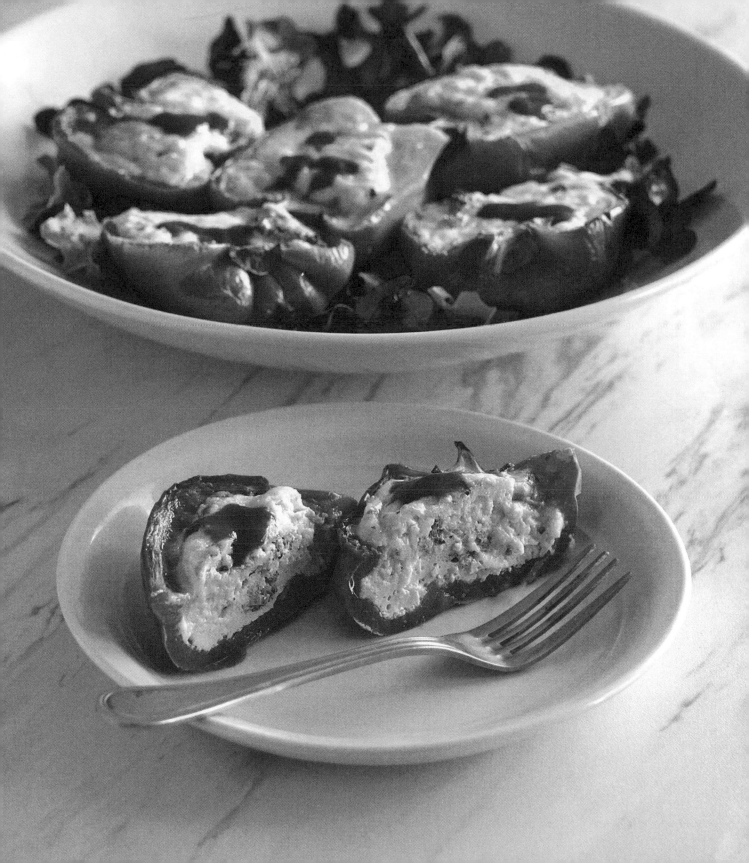

Curried Cauliflower Soup

SERVES 4

Per Serving:

Calories	239
Fat	19g
Protein	4g
Sodium	839mg
Fiber	6g
Carbohydrates	13g
Net Carbs	7g
Sugar	5g

This soup is a light but filling dish made with warming spices. If you're making this soup on one of your higher-carb days, add some chopped carrots with the onions and garlic for a little added sweetness.

2 tablespoons curry powder

1 teaspoon granulated garlic

½ teaspoon ground cumin

½ teaspoon paprika

½ teaspoon sea salt

4 cups riced cauliflower

2 tablespoons plus 2 teaspoons olive oil, divided

½ cup chopped peeled red onion

2 teaspoons minced garlic

2 cups chopped kale

4 cups vegetable broth

1 cup full-fat coconut milk

½ teaspoon crushed red pepper

½ teaspoon ground black pepper

1 Preheat oven to 400°F. Line a baking sheet with parchment paper.

2 Combine curry powder, granulated garlic, cumin, paprika, and salt in a small bowl and mix well. Coat cauliflower rice with 2 tablespoons olive oil and add spices to cauliflower. Toss to coat.

3 Spread cauliflower rice on prepared baking sheet and bake 15 minutes. Remove from oven and set aside.

4 Add remaining olive oil to a large stockpot. Add red onion and minced garlic and cook for 2 minutes over medium heat. Add remaining ingredients and roasted cauliflower and stir to combine.

5 Bring to a light boil and reduce heat to low. Simmer for 30 minutes.

6 Remove from heat, allow to cool slightly, and serve.

Mushroom Risotto

(VG)

The nutritional yeast gives this Mushroom Risotto a creamy, cheesy flavor similar to that of traditional risotto, but if you're sensitive to yeast or you eat dairy, you can replace it with the same amount of grated Parmesan cheese.

2 tablespoons grass-fed butter

2 teaspoons minced garlic

1 small yellow onion, peeled and finely chopped

5 cups sliced cremini mushrooms

1½ tablespoons coconut aminos

1 (12-ounce) bag frozen riced cauliflower

1 cup full-fat coconut milk

1 cup vegetable broth

¼ cup nutritional yeast

¾ teaspoon sea salt

½ teaspoon ground black pepper

½ teaspoon Trader Joe's Mushroom & Company Multipurpose Umami Seasoning Blend

½ teaspoon dried parsley

2 teaspoons arrowroot powder

SERVES 4	
Per Serving:	
Calories	316
Fat	24g
Protein	8g
Sodium	755mg
Fiber	4g
Carbohydrates	17g
Net Carbs	13g
Sugar	8g

NUTRITIONAL YEAST?

Nutritional yeast is made from a type of yeast called *Saccharomyces cerevisiae*. It's similar to the yeast used in baking, but the major difference is in the processing. Nutritional yeast undergoes an intense heating and drying process that basically kills it, so it's not an active form. It's dairy-free, gluten-free, low-carb, and vegan-friendly. When added to foods, it gives the dish a nutty or cheesy flavor. Because of that, it's often used in vegan "cheese" sauces. Note: Nutritional yeast is *not* the same thing as brewer's yeast.

1 Add butter to pot of a pressure cooker and set to the sauté function. When butter is hot, add garlic, onion, and mushrooms and cook until softened, about 7 minutes.

2 Stir in coconut aminos and cook for another 3 minutes, scraping the bottom of the pan with a wooden spoon to remove any browned bits.

3 Add riced cauliflower, coconut milk, broth, nutritional yeast, salt, pepper, umami blend, and parsley. Stir to combine.

4 Seal and cook on manual for 2 minutes. Release pressure manually immediately after cooking.

5 When pressure is released, open lid and stir in arrowroot powder. Let sit for 4 minutes or until thickened, stirring occasionally.

6 Serve warm.

Baked Stuffed Artichokes

(VG)

SERVES 2

Per Serving:

Calories	1,088
Fat	100g
Protein	31g
Sodium	1,530mg
Fiber	15g
Carbohydrates	34g
Net Carbs	19g
Sugar	8g

One large artichoke contains only 8.25 grams of net carbs, making it a good choice for your low-carb keto days. Artichokes also contain prebiotics—meaning they feed the good bacteria in your gut and contribute to gut health.

2 large artichokes

2 cups coarse almond meal

2 teaspoons Italian seasoning

3 tablespoons Parmesan cheese

1 teaspoon garlic salt

½ teaspoon ground black pepper

¼ teaspoon crushed red pepper

¼ cup olive oil

1 tablespoon lemon juice

2 tablespoons butter-flavored coconut oil, melted

½ cup water

1 Preheat oven to 375°F.

2 Lightly pull artichoke leaves to loosen. Slice off stems so artichokes sit flat. Use kitchen scissors to cut off sharp points on tips of leaves.

3 Combine almond meal, Italian seasoning, Parmesan cheese, garlic salt, black pepper, and red pepper in a small bowl and stir to mix well.

4 Add olive oil and lemon juice to almond meal mixture and stir until mixture is moistened and starts to clump.

5 Sprinkle crumb mixture into each leaf of each artichoke. Drizzle with melted coconut oil. Arrange artichokes in an 8" × 8" baking dish.

6 Pour ½ cup water into pan and bake for 75 minutes or until you can easily pull one of the leaves from the artichoke.

7 Allow to cool slightly, then serve.

Spaghetti Squash "Alfredo"

This dish is served cold, but you can combine the squash with the sauce in a saucepan and stir over low heat until heated through.

½ cup raw cashews, soaked

2 tablespoons lemon juice

3 tablespoons nutritional yeast

2 teaspoons coconut aminos

2 cloves garlic

¼ teaspoon sea salt

1 teaspoon onion powder

⅓ cup water

2 cups cooked spaghetti squash

SERVES 2	
Per Serving:	
Calories	236
Fat	13g
Protein	9g
Sodium	389mg
Fiber	4g
Carbohydrates	24g
Net Carbs	20g
Sugar	7g

1 Combine cashews, lemon juice, nutritional yeast, coconut aminos, garlic, salt, onion powder, and water in a food processor and process until smooth.

2 Divide spaghetti squash into two bowls and top each bowl with equal parts of cashew sauce. Serve immediately.

Olive Tapenade

Traditionally, olive tapenade is made with anchovies, but you won't miss them in this vegan version that packs a huge flavor punch.

3 tablespoons olive oil, divided

½ cup cubed eggplant

4 cloves garlic

1 cup pitted Mediterranean olive mix

2 tablespoons capers

3 tablespoons chopped fresh parsley

2 tablespoons lemon juice

¼ teaspoon ground black pepper

SERVES 6	
Per Serving:	
Calories	118
Fat	12g
Protein	0g
Sodium	491mg
Fiber	0g
Carbohydrates	3g
Net Carbs	3g
Sugar	0g

1 Heat 1 tablespoon oil in a medium skillet over medium heat. Add eggplant and cook until softened, about 7 minutes, stirring occasionally. Transfer to a food processor and add remaining ingredients. Pulse until finely chopped, about 1 minute.

2 Remove from food processor and transfer to an airtight container. Store in the refrigerator for up to 5 days until ready to eat.

VE **VG**

Creamed Kale Soup

SERVES 6	
Per Serving:	
Calories	107
Fat	6g
Protein	3g
Sodium	612mg
Fiber	3g
Carbohydrates	9g
Net Carbs	6g
Sugar	4g

This soup gives you a nutritional boost of vitamins A and C, calcium, and potassium, thanks to the kale. If you eat cheese, a tablespoon or so of grated Parmesan cheese sprinkled on top of this Creamed Kale Soup right before serving adds a sharp nuttiness and finishes it off nicely.

2 tablespoons butter-flavored coconut oil

2 teaspoons minced garlic

3 small shallots, peeled and minced

1 large head cauliflower, cut into florets

2 cups chopped kale

4½ cups vegetable broth

1 cup full-fat coconut milk

½ teaspoon sea salt

¼ teaspoon ground black pepper

⅛ teaspoon cayenne pepper

1   Heat coconut oil in a large stockpot over medium heat. Add garlic and shallots and cook for 2 minutes.

2   Add cauliflower to pot and cook until softened, about 6 minutes. Stir in kale and cook until wilted, about 2 minutes.

3   Stir in vegetable broth and bring to a slow boil over medium-high heat. Cook for 5 more minutes.

4   Reduce heat to low and use an immersion blender to purée soup. Stir in coconut milk, salt, black pepper, and cayenne pepper. Cook for another 2 minutes, remove from heat, and serve warm.

One-Pan Taco Skillet

This vegan One-Pan Taco Skillet is bursting with Mexican flavor and vegetables. Everyone will be asking for seconds.

3 tablespoons olive oil

1 small yellow onion, peeled and diced

1 medium green bell pepper, seeded and diced

1 small red mini sweet pepper, seeded and diced

1 small eggplant, diced

1 large zucchini, diced

1 cup riced cauliflower

½ cup walnuts, finely chopped

½ cup petite-diced tomatoes, drained

1 (4-ounce) can green chilis

2 tablespoons keto-friendly taco seasoning

¼ cup water

1 Heat olive oil in a medium skillet over medium heat. Add onion and cook for 2 minutes.

2 Stir in bell pepper and mini red pepper and cook for another 4 minutes. Add eggplant, zucchini, and riced cauliflower and cook until softened, stirring occasionally, about 10 minutes.

3 Stir in walnuts, tomatoes, and green chilis. Add taco seasoning and water and stir until incorporated.

4 Reduce heat to low and let simmer for 5 minutes or until moisture has evaporated. Remove from heat and serve.

SERVES 4	
Per Serving:	
Calories	282
Fat	21g
Protein	6g
Sodium	1,002mg
Fiber	10g
Carbohydrates	23g
Net Carbs	13g
Sugar	11g

HOMEMADE TACO SEASONING

You can make your own taco seasoning at home. Once you try it, you'll probably prefer to make it over purchasing those seasoning packets. To make it, combine 1 tablespoon chili powder, 1½ teaspoons ground cumin, ½ teaspoon paprika, ¼ teaspoon dried oregano, ¼ teaspoon crushed red pepper, ¼ teaspoon garlic powder, ¼ teaspoon onion powder, 1 teaspoon salt, and 1 teaspoon ground black pepper.

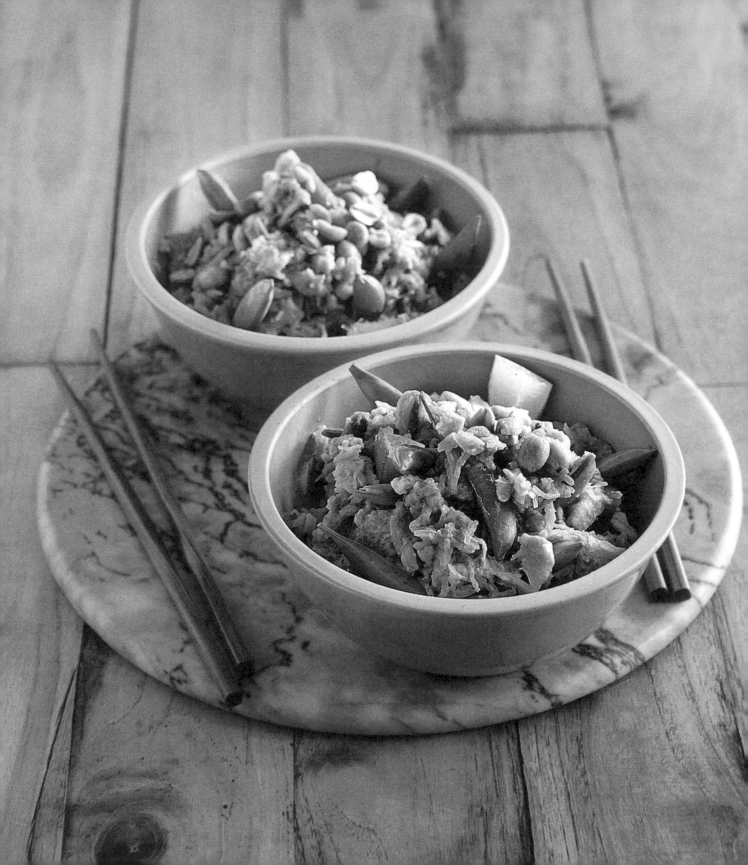

Vegetarian Pad Thai

(VG)

If you're enjoying this Vegetarian Pad Thai on one of your higher-carb days, you can add a couple cups of sugar snap peas into the recipe when you cook the onions. If you want to make it a vegan dish, omit the eggs.

4 tablespoons lime juice

2 teaspoons minced garlic

1 teaspoon crushed red pepper

2 tablespoons coconut aminos, divided

1 teaspoon minced fresh ginger

1 teaspoon rice vinegar

1 tablespoon golden monk fruit sweetener

½ cup no-sugar-added peanut butter

½ cup full-fat coconut milk

3 large eggs

2 tablespoons butter-flavored coconut oil

1 medium yellow onion, peeled and sliced thinly

3 tablespoons chopped peanuts

4 cups cooked spaghetti squash

SERVES 4	
Per Serving:	
Calories	520
Fat	41g
Protein	17g
Sodium	236mg
Fiber	10g
Carbohydrates	26g
Net Carbs	13g
Sugar	10g

1 Combine lime juice, garlic, red pepper, 1 tablespoon coconut aminos, ginger, rice vinegar, monk fruit sweetener, and peanut butter in a food processor and process until smooth, about 1 minute. Pulse in coconut milk until smooth, another 30 seconds. Set aside.

2 Combine remaining coconut aminos and eggs in a small bowl and whisk to mix.

3 Heat coconut oil in a medium skillet over medium heat. Add egg mixture and scramble until eggs are done, about 3 minutes. Remove eggs from heat and set aside.

4 Add onion to pan and cook until softened, about 4 minutes. Add peanuts and cook for another 2 minutes.

5 Add spaghetti squash and stir until everything is combined. Pour peanut sauce over spaghetti squash, add cooked eggs, and toss to coat.

6 Remove from heat and serve warm.

VE **VG**

Coconut Thai Zoodle Soup

SERVES 4

Per Serving:

Calories	207
Fat	13g
Protein	5g
Sodium	1,107mg
Fiber	4g
Carbohydrates	19g
Net Carbs	15g
Sugar	12g

If you want to enjoy this soup on one of your high-carb days, you can replace the zucchini noodles with sweet potato noodles or butternut squash noodles to add some complex carbohydrates to it. If you're not vegan, you can use grass-fed heavy cream or half-and-half in place of the coconut cream.

1 tablespoon coconut oil

2 tablespoons red curry paste

1 tablespoon red chili paste

1 teaspoon ground curry powder

1 teaspoon ground coriander

2 cups vegetable broth

1 tablespoon coconut aminos

½ cup chopped peeled red onion

1 (15-ounce) can full-fat coconut milk

3 large zucchini, spiralized

1 tablespoon fresh lime juice

¼ cup fresh cilantro

1 Heat coconut oil in a medium stockpot over medium-high heat. Add curry paste and chili paste and cook for 1 minute. Add curry powder and coriander and cook for another minute.

2 Add vegetable broth, coconut aminos, and onion. Bring to a slow boil and then reduce heat and simmer for 15 minutes. Stir in coconut milk and allow to heat through, about 2 minutes.

3 Stir in zucchini and cook until softened, but still slightly crisp, about 3 minutes. Remove from heat and stir in lime juice and cilantro.

4 Serve immediately.

Spinach and Artichoke Dip

Skip store-bought versions of this dip—this keto-friendly version tastes better anyway. Raw zucchini slices make the perfect accompaniment for this Spinach and Artichoke Dip, which is rich in mono-unsaturated fats and antioxidants.

1 (10-ounce) package frozen chopped spinach, thawed and squeezed dry

2 large avocados, peeled, cut in half, and pitted

2 garlic cloves

¼ cup fresh parsley

¾ cup full-fat coconut yogurt

1 tablespoon lime juice

3 tablespoons olive oil

½ teaspoon sea salt

¼ teaspoon crushed red pepper

1 (9-ounce) package frozen artichoke hearts, thawed and chopped

1 Combine all ingredients, except artichoke hearts, in a food processor. Process until smooth.

2 Transfer mixture to a medium bowl and stir in chopped artichoke hearts.

3 Serve immediately or store in an airtight container in the refrigerator until ready to eat, up to 1 week.

SERVES 12

Per Serving:

Calories	117
Fat	9g
Protein	2g
Sodium	150mg
Fiber	5g
Carbohydrates	8g
Net Carbs	3g
Sugar	2g

(VE) (VG) **Pan-Fried Walnut Cabbage**

SERVES 2

Per Serving:

Calories	494
Fat	41g
Protein	10g
Sodium	964mg
Fiber	8g
Carbohydrates	26g
Net Carbs	18g
Sugar	13g

YOUR BRAIN ON WALNUTS

Your brain is composed of about 60 percent fat. Walnuts contain about 65 percent fat. Approximately 8 to 14 percent of the fat in walnuts is in the form of alpha-linolenic acid, or ALA—a polyunsaturated fat that helps reduce inflammation and gets converted to docosahexaenoic acid (DHA), which is essential for brain health. Eating good fats provides your brain with the fat it needs to create new brain cells and one of the major structures of every cell in your body, called the *phospholipid bilayer*.

Walnuts are loaded with antioxidants and are rich in a specific omega-3 fatty acid called alpha-linolenic acid, *or ALA, which is good for your heart. No other nuts contain significant amounts of ALA.*

1 tablespoon avocado oil

1 medium white onion, peeled and chopped

2 teaspoons minced garlic

4 cups shredded green cabbage

1 teaspoon red chili paste

1 teaspoon apple cider vinegar

2 tablespoons coconut aminos

1 tablespoon no-sugar-added creamy peanut butter

1 tablespoon sesame oil

½ cup chopped walnuts

1 tablespoon sesame seeds

1 Heat avocado oil in a medium skillet over medium heat. Add onion and cook for 2 minutes. Stir in garlic and cook for an additional minute.

2 Add cabbage, chili paste, vinegar, coconut aminos, peanut butter, and sesame oil and stir to combine. Cover and cook for 6 minutes or until cabbage starts to soften.

3 Stir in walnuts, cover, and cook for another 5 minutes. Remove from heat and sprinkle sesame seeds on top.

4 Serve warm.

Vegetable-Loaded Soup

(VG)

The more variety you have in your vegetable intake, the less likely you are to develop nutrient deficiencies. This Vegetable-Loaded Soup is bursting with vitamins, minerals, and antioxidants that supply your body with everything you need to stay healthy. To make this soup vegan, you can use nutritional yeast in place of the Parmesan cheese.

SERVES 6	
Per Serving:	
Calories	116
Fat	4g
Protein	5g
Sodium	1,012mg
Fiber	5g
Carbohydrates	15g
Net Carbs	10g
Sugar	7g

1 tablespoon butter-flavored coconut oil

2 teaspoons minced garlic

1 large yellow onion, peeled and diced

1 teaspoon sea salt

½ teaspoon ground black pepper

2 tablespoons tomato paste

2 cups chopped green cabbage

2 cups cauliflower florets

1 medium carrot, peeled and finely chopped

3 medium celery stalks, cut into half-moons

1 medium green bell pepper, seeded and diced

1 (15-ounce) can fire-roasted diced tomatoes, drained

4 cups vegetable broth

1 teaspoon dried parsley

1 teaspoon dried basil

½ teaspoon dried thyme

½ teaspoon paprika

¼ teaspoon ground cumin

¼ cup grated Parmesan cheese

1   Heat coconut oil in a large stockpot over medium heat. Add garlic and onion and cook for 1 minute. Sprinkle salt and pepper and stir. Cook for another 5 minutes.

2   Stir in tomato paste and cook for an additional minute. Add remaining ingredients, except Parmesan cheese, and stir to combine.

3   Reduce heat to low and simmer for 1 hour.

4   Transfer 1 cup of soup to a blender and blend until smooth. Stir puréed soup back into stockpot.

5   Simmer for 15 more minutes. Remove from heat and sprinkle with Parmesan cheese before serving.

Cauliflower Cashew Tikka Masala

WHAT IS HARISSA PASTE?

A staple in North African and Middle Eastern cooking, harissa paste combines dried chilis, garlic, olive oil, and various toasted spices, like cumin, coriander, caraway, and paprika. The heat level varies depending on the type of chilis used, but it's generally pretty hot. You can find harissa paste in a jar, can, or tube in the international foods section of your grocery store. Most of them are keto-friendly, but double-check your labels just in case!

The harissa paste used in this recipe makes this Cauliflower Cashew Tikka Masala quite spicy. If you don't want the extra heat, scale it back or omit it and use chili powder instead.

2 tablespoons butter-flavored coconut oil

1 medium yellow onion, peeled and diced

2 teaspoons minced garlic

¼ teaspoon ground ginger

2 teaspoons garam masala

1 teaspoon curry powder

2 teaspoons harissa paste

¼ teaspoon ground cumin

1 teaspoon sea salt

1 (28-ounce) can petite-diced tomatoes with liquid

1 tablespoon monk fruit-sweetened maple syrup

4 cups riced cauliflower

½ cup full-fat coconut milk

1 tablespoon lemon juice

½ cup cashews

¼ cup chopped fresh cilantro

1 Turn pressure cooker on to sauté function. Add coconut oil to pot. Once oil is hot, add onion and garlic and cook for 3 minutes or until onions start to soften. Stir in ginger, garam masala, curry powder, harissa paste, cumin, and salt. Cook for another minute, stirring constantly.

2 Add diced tomatoes (and their juice), maple syrup, and riced cauliflower to pot and stir. Secure lid.

3 Choose the manual setting and set to pressure cook on high for 2 minutes. When timer goes off, release pressure manually.

4 Remove lid and stir in coconut milk and lemon juice.

5 Allow to cool slightly, then serve topped with cashews and cilantro.

Garlic Cheddar Broccoli Spaghetti Squash

(VG)

You won't miss traditional pasta with this hearty dish. This recipe calls for cooked spaghetti squash. You can easily whip up a batch by cutting a spaghetti squash in half, scooping out the seeds, and roasting it, cut side up, at 375°F for about 1 hour.

4 tablespoons butter-flavored coconut oil

2 teaspoons minced garlic

2 medium shallots, peeled and minced

2 tablespoons vegetable broth

1½ cups bite-sized broccoli florets

½ cup grated Parmesan cheese

½ cup shredded Cheddar cheese

2½ cups cooked spaghetti squash

½ teaspoon sea salt

¼ teaspoon ground black pepper

SERVES 4	
Per Serving:	
Calories	334
Fat	28g
Protein	11g
Sodium	861mg
Fiber	2g
Carbohydrates	11g
Net Carbs	9g
Sugar	5g

1 Heat coconut oil in a medium skillet over medium heat. Add garlic and shallots and cook for 2 minutes. Stir in vegetable broth, add broccoli florets, and cover.

2 Reduce heat to low and cook for 6 minutes or until broccoli softens and turns a bright green.

3 Add Parmesan cheese and Cheddar cheese to skillet and stir until melted. Add spaghetti squash, salt, and pepper and stir to combine.

4 Remove from heat and serve immediately.

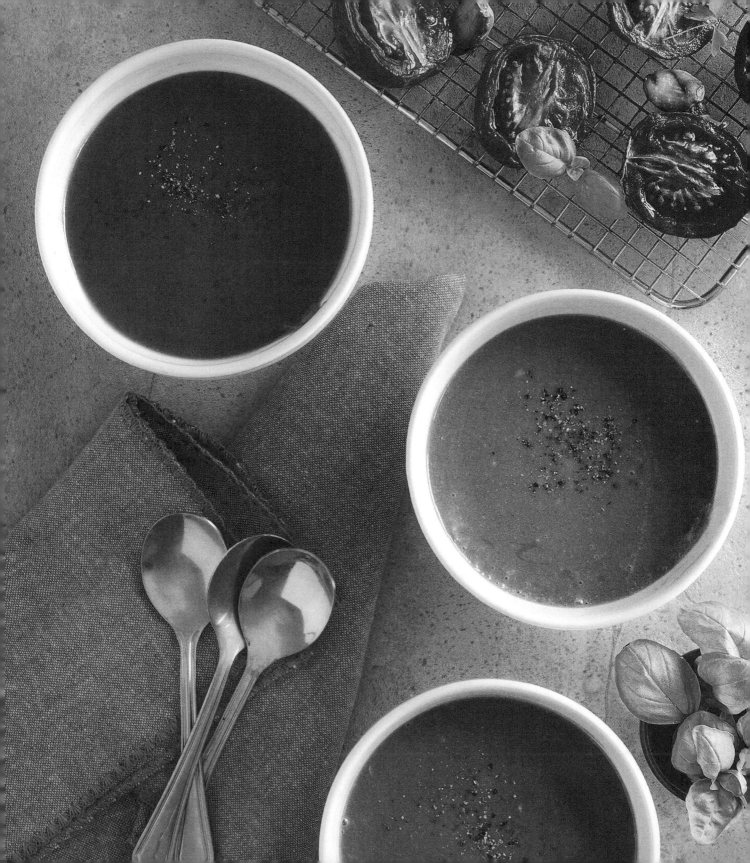

Roasted Tomato and Basil Soup

VE VG

Roasting the tomatoes before using them in this soup deepens their flavor and adds smokiness. If you're short on time and you want to make this soup in a pinch, you can skip the roasting.

Roasted Tomatoes and Garlic

4 pounds fresh Roma tomatoes, cut in half

6 cloves garlic, sliced

2 tablespoons olive oil

1 teaspoon sea salt

½ teaspoon ground black pepper

Tomato Basil Soup

2 tablespoons butter-flavored coconut oil

½ teaspoon crushed red pepper

1 teaspoon onion powder

½ teaspoon ground black pepper

½ teaspoon sea salt

1 cup packed fresh basil leaves

1½ cups vegetable broth

½ cup full-fat coconut milk

SERVES 6

Per Serving:

Calories	175
Fat	13g
Protein	3g
Sodium	327mg
Fiber	4g
Carbohydrates	14g
Net Carbs	10g
Sugar	9g

1 **For Roasted Tomatoes and Garlic:** Preheat oven to 300°F. Line a baking sheet with parchment paper.

2 Combine tomatoes and garlic in a large mixing bowl. Drizzle with olive oil and sprinkle salt and pepper on top. Toss to coat evenly. Arrange tomatoes in a single layer, cut side up, on prepared baking sheet and roast for 90 minutes.

3 **For Tomato Basil Soup:** Remove roasted tomatoes and garlic from oven and transfer (with any juices) to the pot of a pressure cooker.

4 Add all Tomato Basil Soup ingredients, except coconut milk, and stir to combine. Cover and seal pressure cooker.

5 Choose the soup setting and set the timer for 7 minutes. After timer goes off, allow pressure to release naturally. Open lid carefully and use an immersion blender to purée soup to desired consistency. Stir in coconut milk.

6 Allow to cool slightly, then serve.

Chocolate Avocado Pops

SERVES 6

Per Serving:

Calories	416
Fat	34g
Protein	5g
Sodium	15mg
Fiber	9g
Carbohydrates	40g
Net Carbs	18g
Sugar	1g

GO MONOUNSATURATED!

Avocados get a lot of praise for being one of the healthiest fats out there—and for good reason! The fat in avocados is mostly in the form of monounsaturated fat (77 percent of avocados' calories come from fat), which helps reduce inflammation and lowers your risk of developing heart disease. A diet high in monounsaturated fats has also been linked to better blood sugar regulation and lower levels of LDL (or "bad") cholesterol.

Avocado for dessert? Yes, that's right! Avocados make an excellent pop base because they're creamy and full of satisfying fats. Plus, when you mix them with the other ingredients, you can hardly taste them!

3 large ripe avocados, peeled, cut in half, and pitted

2 tablespoons lemon juice

3 tablespoons granulated monk fruit sweetener

¾ cup full-fat coconut milk

1 teaspoon vanilla extract

1 cup vegan stevia-sweetened chocolate chips

1 tablespoon butter-flavored coconut oil

1 Combine avocados, lemon juice, sweetener, coconut milk, and vanilla extract in a food processor. Process until smooth.

2 Pour mixture evenly into a six-mold Popsicle mold. Freeze for 6 hours or until set.

3 Combine chocolate chips and coconut oil in a small saucepan over low heat. Stir until chocolate melts and mixture is smooth. Remove from heat and allow to cool to room temperature.

4 Dip pops in chocolate, allow chocolate to harden, and serve immediately.

Crushed Macadamia Nut Brownies

These brownies taste even better the next day. Their chocolate flavor develops a little more, and they get even fudgier. If you can resist them, allow them to cool completely and enjoy them the day after you make them.

6 tablespoons cold water

2 tablespoons ground flaxseed

1 large avocado, peeled, cut in half, and pitted

⅓ cup golden monk fruit sweetener

¼ cup monk fruit–sweetened maple syrup

3 tablespoons butter-flavored coconut oil

1 teaspoon vanilla extract

½ cup unsweetened raw cacao powder

1 teaspoon baking soda

½ teaspoon sea salt

½ cup crushed macadamia nuts

SERVES 9

Per Serving:	
Calories	172
Fat	16g
Protein	3g
Sodium	386mg
Fiber	5g
Carbohydrates	15g
Net Carbs	1g
Sugar	1g

1 Preheat oven to 350°F. Lightly coat an 8" × 8" pan with coconut oil baking spray.

2 Stir water and flaxseed together in a small bowl and mix. Refrigerate for 15 minutes or until mixture thickens.

3 Combine flaxseed mixture, avocado, monk fruit sweetener, maple syrup, coconut oil, and vanilla extract in a food processor. Process until smooth, stopping to scrape down sides of bowl whenever necessary.

4 Add remaining ingredients, except macadamia nuts, and process until smooth, about 1 minute.

5 Add macadamia nuts and pulse once or twice, just to incorporate.

6 Transfer batter to prepared pan and spread evenly with a spatula. Bake for 25 minutes or until a toothpick inserted in the center comes out clean. Remove from oven and allow to cool.

7 Cut into nine brownies and serve.

VE VG

Rich Chocolate Pudding

SERVES 4

Per Serving:

Calories	354
Fat	28g
Protein	5g
Sodium	92mg
Fiber	10g
Carbohydrates	30g
Net Carbs	12g
Sugar	1g

A dessert that's ready in minutes, low in sugar, high in fat, and delicious? Does it get any better? This Rich Chocolate Pudding has the perfect amount of sweetness to stop your sweet tooth and fill you up so you don't reach for those midnight snacks.

½ cup vegan stevia-sweetened chocolate chips

2 teaspoons butter-flavored coconut oil

2 large ripe avocados, peeled, pitted, and roughly chopped

3 tablespoons unsweetened raw cacao powder

1 tablespoon monk fruit–sweetened maple syrup

½ teaspoon finely ground espresso

¼ cup unsweetened chocolate almond milk

1 teaspoon vanilla extract

⅛ teaspoon sea salt

1 Combine chocolate chips and coconut oil in a small saucepan over low heat. Stir constantly until chocolate is melted and mixture is smooth.

2 Transfer melted chocolate to food processor and add remaining ingredients. Process until smooth.

3 Transfer mixture to 4 bowls and serve immediately. Note: If you want a thicker, mousse-like consistency, refrigerate for 2 hours before serving.

CHAPTER 10

Carb-Day Breakfast

Strawberry Banana Yogurt

SERVES 1	
Per Serving:	
Calories	256
Fat	15g
Protein	11g
Sodium	101mg
Fiber	2g
Carbohydrates	22g
Net Carbs	20g
Sugar	13g

Make sure you're getting yogurt that's full-fat and plain. Most sweetened, flavored yogurt contains too many carbs (and too many undesirable ingredients) even for your high-carb days.

1 (5.3-ounce) container plain full-fat yogurt

1 tablespoon no-sugar-added peanut butter, melted

½ teaspoon vanilla extract

2 tablespoons mashed peeled ripe banana

2 tablespoons chopped strawberries

2 teaspoons stevia-sweetened maple syrup

1 Combine all ingredients in a small bowl and stir with a spoon until incorporated.

2 Serve immediately.

Chocolate-Covered Cherry Smoothie

SERVES 1	
Per Serving:	
Calories	366
Fat	27g
Protein	13g
Sodium	261mg
Fiber	8g
Carbohydrates	27g
Net Carbs	19g
Sugar	11g

The bananas and cherries give this Chocolate-Covered Cherry Smoothie the perfect amount of sweetness to satisfy even the most intense of chocolate cravings. It still uses high-quality ingredients and sneaks in some spinach!

¾ cup unsweetened chocolate almond milk

2 tablespoons banana milk

1 tablespoon unsweetened cocoa powder

3 raw Brazil nuts

1 teaspoon melted coconut oil

6 frozen pitted dark cherries

½ medium peeled banana, frozen

1 tablespoon chocolate MCT oil powder

½ cup frozen chopped spinach

1 tablespoon grass-fed collagen powder

1 Combine all ingredients in a blender.

2 Blend until smooth. Serve immediately.

Fried Rice Patties

These patties come together quickly and are full of flavor. Pair these Fried Rice Patties with some over-easy eggs and a side of bacon for a hearty, high-carb breakfast.

1 cup cooked short-grain brown rice

4 slices cooked no-sugar-added bacon, chopped

½ cup chopped peeled yellow onion

¼ cup shredded Cheddar cheese

1 tablespoon grated Parmesan cheese

1 large egg, lightly whisked

1 tablespoon coconut flour

1 tablespoon arrowroot flour

¼ teaspoon sea salt

¼ teaspoon ground black pepper

¼ teaspoon crushed red pepper

¼ teaspoon garlic powder

¼ teaspoon dried minced onion

2 tablespoons butter-flavored coconut oil

SERVES 4	
Per Serving:	
Calories	245
Fat	15g
Protein	9g
Sodium	405mg
Fiber	2g
Carbohydrates	18g
Net Carbs	16g
Sugar	1g

1 Combine all ingredients, except coconut oil, in a medium bowl and mix well to incorporate.

2 Divide mixture into four equal portions and flatten into patties.

3 Heat coconut oil in a large skillet over medium-high heat. Add patties to hot pan and cook for 5 minutes. Flip, then cook for another 5 minutes or until golden brown.

4 Remove from heat and serve warm.

Sweet Potato Fritters

Like zucchini, sweet potatoes have a high moisture content, so allowing them to sweat for 30 minutes before incorporating them into certain recipes will help prevent sogginess. Don't skip this important step.

SERVES 2

Per Serving:	
Calories	407
Fat	22g
Protein	11g
Sodium	660mg
Fiber	16g
Carbohydrates	43g
Net Carbs	27g
Sugar	5g

THE SWEET CHOICE

Sweet potatoes are high in carbohydrates, but they have a low glycemic index, so those carbohydrates are metabolized by the body slowly, making them a good choice for a carb source on your high-carb days. More than that, research shows that sweet potatoes can increase the hormone adiponectin, which helps release fatty acids from fat cells so your body can use them for whatever it needs.

1 medium sweet potato, peeled

½ teaspoon sea salt

2½ tablespoons coconut flour

2 tablespoons arrowroot powder

1 large egg, lightly beaten

½ teaspoon onion powder

½ teaspoon garlic powder

½ teaspoon ground black pepper

2 tablespoons butter-flavored coconut oil

1 Shred sweet potato using a cheese grater or the shredding attachment of a food processor. Transfer sweet potato to a strainer and sprinkle with salt. Toss to coat. Let sweet potato sit for 30 minutes to let excess water drain out.

2 After 30 minutes, use a cheesecloth or a nut milk bag to squeeze out as much excess moisture as you can.

3 Combine remaining ingredients, except coconut oil, in a medium bowl and stir to combine. Add sweet potato and stir well.

4 Heat coconut oil in a medium skillet over medium heat. Scoop sweet potato mixture by the tablespoonful into hot skillet. Press down to flatten into rounds. Repeat until skillet is full. Cook for 3 minutes or until fritters start to brown. Flip and cook on the other side for another 3 minutes.

5 Place fritters on paper towel–lined plate to absorb excess oil.

6 Repeat until all fritters are cooked. Serve immediately.

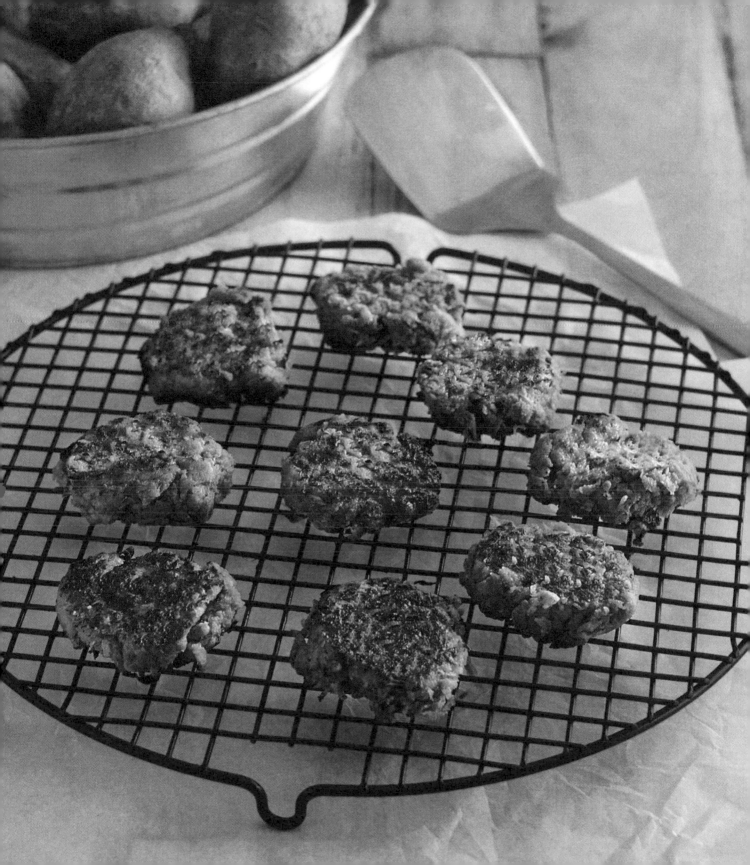

Sweet Potato Home Fries

SERVES 4	
Per Serving:	
Calories	478
Fat	45g
Protein	2g
Sodium	546mg
Fiber	3g
Carbohydrates	21g
Net Carbs	18g
Sugar	7g

Make these Sweet Potato Home Fries a complete carb-day breakfast by adding over-easy eggs, a side of no-sugar-added bacon, and a heap of your favorite vegetables to your plate.

3 tablespoons butter-flavored coconut oil

2 large sweet potatoes, peeled and cubed

1 teaspoon sea salt

1 teaspoon ground black pepper

1 teaspoon paprika

1/16 teaspoon crushed red pepper

1 Heat oil in a medium skillet over medium-high heat. When oil is hot, add potatoes to pan.

2 Cook for 2 minutes, stir, and cook for an additional 2 minutes. Sprinkle seasonings on top and stir to combine.

3 Allow potatoes to cook for another 5 minutes without stirring. Stir and then continue cooking for 5 minutes or until potatoes are crisp on the outside and soft on the inside.

4 Remove from heat and serve hot.

Butternut Squash Breakfast Bowls

If you want to save time down the road, double or triple the amount you make and store it in the refrigerator (for up to 1 week) until you're ready to top it with an egg and the rest of your ingredients.

2 cups cubed butternut squash

1 tablespoon olive oil

1 teaspoon garlic powder

¼ teaspoon ground cumin

¼ teaspoon paprika

1 teaspoon sea salt, divided

1 teaspoon ground black pepper, divided

⅛ teaspoon ground cinnamon

1 tablespoon grass-fed butter

1 teaspoon minced garlic

¼ cup chopped peeled yellow onion

1 cup chopped kale

4 large eggs, whisked

1 large avocado, peeled, pitted, and chopped

½ cup crumbled feta cheese

SERVES 2	
Per Serving:	
Calories	575
Fat	42g
Protein	22g
Sodium	1,460mg
Fiber	12g
Carbohydrates	31g
Net Carbs	19g
Sugar	5g

1 Preheat oven to 425°F. Line a baking sheet with parchment paper.

2 Combine butternut squash, olive oil, garlic powder, cumin, paprika, ½ teaspoon salt, ½ teaspoon pepper, and cinnamon in a medium mixing bowl. Toss to coat.

3 Spread butternut squash on baking sheet in a single layer. Roast for 10 minutes, flip squash, then roast another 15 minutes or until butternut squash is tender and starting to crisp on the edges. Remove from oven and divide evenly into two bowls.

4 Heat butter in a medium skillet over medium heat. Add minced garlic and cook for 1 minute. Add onion and cook until softened, about 5 minutes. Stir in kale and cook until wilted, about 2 minutes.

5 Add eggs and remaining salt and pepper to mixture and scramble until egg is cooked through, about 4 minutes. Remove from heat and put equal amounts of egg mixture on top of each bowl of butternut squash.

6 Top each bowl with ½ avocado and ¼ cup feta cheese.

Blueberry Banana Mug Muffin

SERVES 1

Per Serving:

Calories	222
Fat	13g
Protein	11g
Sodium	357mg
Fiber	5g
Carbohydrates	40g
Net Carbs	11g
Sugar	4g

A WILD CARBOHYDRATE CHOICE

Wild blueberries are loaded with purple pigments called *anthocyanins*, antioxidants that have been shown to help reduce brain inflammation and repair the structure of the blood-brain barrier, which protects the brain and spinal cord from foreign invaders. Wild blueberries contain more anthocyanins than regular blueberries because of the stress they're put under while growing. They have about 9 grams per ½ cup, 6 grams of which come from fiber.

This Blueberry Banana Mug Muffin is ready in under 5 minutes if you cook it in the microwave. If you prefer not to use a microwave, you can mix the ingredients in an oven-safe ramekin and then bake at 350°F for 11 minutes or until muffin sets.

2 tablespoons almond flour

1 tablespoon coconut flour

2 tablespoons golden monk fruit sweetener

½ teaspoon baking powder

¼ teaspoon ground cinnamon

¼ teaspoon vanilla extract

1 large egg

1½ tablespoons mashed peeled banana

2 tablespoons unsweetened vanilla almond milk

3 tablespoons frozen wild blueberries

1 Combine all ingredients, except blueberries, in a microwave-safe mug and whisk until incorporated. Stir in blueberries.

2 Microwave for 45 seconds and check for doneness. If muffin isn't done, cook in 15-second intervals until set.

3 Let cool slightly and then serve.

Sweet Potato Casserole

This Sweet Potato Casserole combines everything—healthy carbo-hydrates, protein, and fat—all in one pan. If you're using it for meal prep, take what you need and freeze the rest in portions for up to 6 months for an easy breakfast on your next high-carb day.

½ pound no-sugar-added pork breakfast sausage

2 cups shredded sweet potatoes

2 tablespoons grass-fed butter, melted

¼ teaspoon paprika

1 cup shredded Cheddar cheese

1 cup Monterey Jack cheese

¼ cup minced peeled shallots

½ cup chopped kale

1 (8-ounce) container full-fat cottage cheese

8 large eggs, whisked

SERVES 6	
Per Serving:	
Calories	414
Fat	32g
Protein	25g
Sodium	750mg
Fiber	1g
Carbohydrates	8g
Net Carbs	7g
Sugar	3g

1 Preheat oven to 375°F.

2 Heat a medium skillet over medium heat. Crumble sausage into pan and cook until no longer pink, about 7 minutes. Set aside.

3 Combine sweet potatoes, butter, and paprika in a medium bowl and stir to mix. Transfer mixture to a 9" × 9" baking dish and spread in an even layer.

4 Transfer sausage to a medium bowl and add remaining ingredients. Stir to combine.

5 Pour egg mixture over sweet potato layer and spread out evenly.

6 Bake for 1 hour or until eggs are set. Remove from heat and allow to cool slightly before serving.

Banana Quinoa Porridge

This Banana Quinoa Porridge has a texture similar to that of rice pudding. After cooking, top it with your favorite keto-friendly mix-ins. Crushed walnuts, berries, shaved coconut, and stevia-sweetened chocolate chips are great choices.

SERVES 4

Per Serving:

Calories	246
Fat	14g
Protein	5g
Sodium	171mg
Fiber	3g
Carbohydrates	27g
Net Carbs	18g
Sugar	7g

QUINOA AS A CARBOHYDRATE SOURCE

Although it's often classified as a grain, quinoa is really a seed that comes from the quinoa plant. It's one of the few plant-based foods that contains all of the nine essential amino acids, making it an excellent carbohydrate source for your high-carb days. One cup of cooked quinoa contains about 39 grams of carbohydrates, about 5 grams of which come from fiber.

½ cup sprouted quinoa, rinsed

1 cup water

1 large ripe banana, peeled

1 cup full-fat coconut milk

⅓ cup grass-fed half-and-half

2 tablespoons monk fruit–sweetened maple syrup

2 teaspoons grass-fed butter

½ teaspoon ground cinnamon

⅛ teaspoon ground nutmeg

¼ teaspoon sea salt

1　Combine quinoa and water in a medium saucepan and let sit for 30 minutes. After 30 minutes, turn heat to high and bring mixture to a boil. Reduce heat to low, cover, and simmer for 15 minutes or until water is absorbed.

2　While quinoa is cooking, combine remaining ingredients in a food processor and process until smooth.

3　Stir banana mixture into quinoa and increase heat to medium. Cook, stirring frequently, for 10 minutes or until porridge thickens.

4　Remove from heat and serve warm.

Butternut Squash Breakfast Skillet

Have extra vegetables you want to use? This Butternut Squash Breakfast Skillet is a great way to do it. Although the recipe calls for onion and kale, you can add any extra vegetables that you want to it.

2 tablespoons grass-fed butter

2 cups cubed butternut squash

½ medium yellow onion, peeled and diced

1 pound no-sugar-added ground sage pork breakfast sausage

2 teaspoons minced garlic

1 teaspoon dried rosemary

¼ teaspoon crushed red pepper

2 cups chopped kale

4 large eggs

1 teaspoon sea salt

½ teaspoon ground black pepper

1 Preheat oven to 350°F.

2 Heat butter in a medium cast iron skillet over medium-high heat. Add butternut squash and cook for 5 minutes or until it starts to soften. Add onions and cook for another 3 minutes.

3 Crumble breakfast sausage into pan and cook until sausage is no longer pink, about 7 more minutes.

4 Stir in garlic, rosemary, red pepper, and kale and cook, stirring occasionally, until kale wilts, about 3 minutes.

5 Form four wells in butternut squash mixture for the eggs. Crack an egg into each well and transfer skillet to preheated oven.

6 Bake for 15 minutes or until eggs set.

7 Remove from oven and sprinkle salt and pepper on top. Serve immediately.

SERVES 4	
Per Serving:	
Calories	390
Fat	30g
Protein	18g
Sodium	1,054mg
Fiber	2g
Carbohydrates	12g
Net Carbs	10g
Sugar	3g

FALLING IN LOVE WITH BUTTERNUT SQUASH

In general, eating produce is linked to a reduced risk of heart disease—but yellow and orange vegetables, like butternut squash, may be particularly helpful. According to a study published in the journal *Scientific Reports* in 2016, each daily serving of yellow-orange vegetables that you eat drops your risk of heart disease by as much as 23 percent.

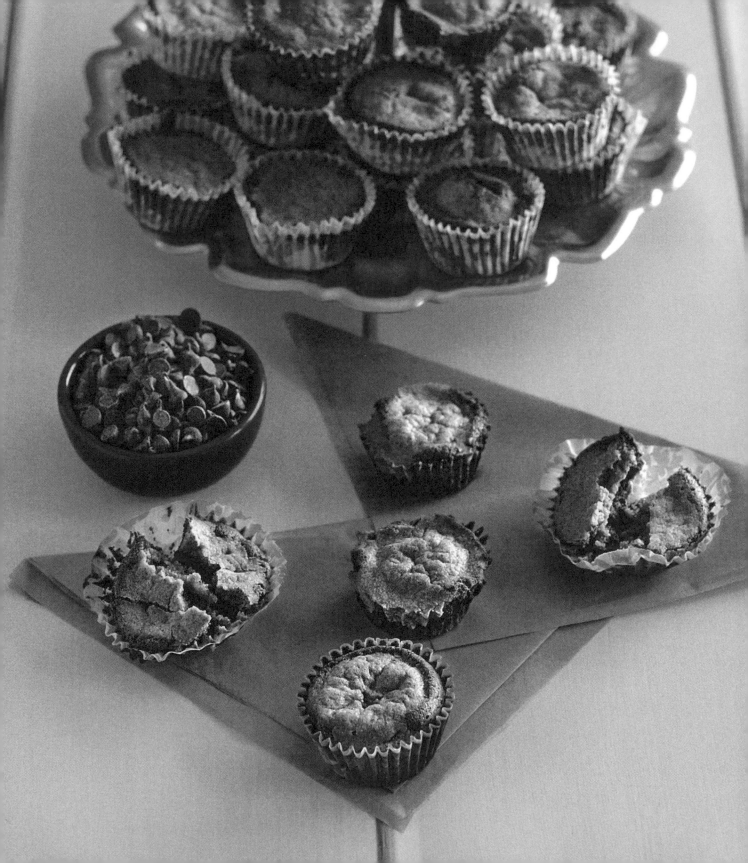

Chocolate Pumpkin Mini Muffins

These Chocolate Pumpkin Mini Muffins aren't just delicious; they're also good for you. Unlike regular muffins, which are loaded with sugar and not much else, these contain fiber, beta-carotene, starch, and antioxidants.

¼ cup cassava flour

2 tablespoons paleo flour

¼ teaspoon baking powder

¼ teaspoon sea salt

⅓ cup grass-fed butter, melted

¾ cup granulated monk fruit sweetener

1 teaspoon vanilla extract

2 large eggs

2 tablespoons unsweetened cocoa powder

¼ cup stevia-sweetened chocolate chips

¼ cup pumpkin purée

¾ teaspoon pumpkin pie spice

SERVES 8 (MAKES 24 MUFFINS)	
Per Serving:	
Calories	156
Fat	12g
Protein	3g
Sodium	84mg
Fiber	2g
Carbohydrates	12g
Net Carbs	1g
Sugar	1g

1 Preheat oven to 350°F. Line a mini muffin tin with paper or silicone liners.

2 Combine cassava flour, paleo flour, baking powder, and salt in a medium mixing bowl.

3 Add butter, monk fruit sweetener, and vanilla to another medium bowl and beat with a handheld mixer until smooth. Beat in eggs one at a time.

4 Fold flour mixture into wet ingredients and stir until incorporated. Divide mixture between two bowls.

5 Stir cocoa powder and chocolate chips into one bowl. Add remaining ingredients to the other bowl and stir until smooth.

6 Using a 1.25" cookie scoop, scoop equal amounts of chocolate mixture into each well of the muffin tin. When chocolate mixture is gone, scoop equal amounts of pumpkin mixture on top of chocolate mixture.

7 Bake for 25 minutes or until a toothpick inserted in the center comes out clean. Remove from oven and allow to cool. Remove from muffin tin and serve.

THE SCOOP ON CASSAVA FLOUR

Cassava flour is a gluten-free, grain-free alternative to wheat flour that comes from the root of the cassava plant. It has a mild, neutral taste and fine texture that blends in well in baked goods. Unlike other gluten-free flours, you can use cassava flour in place of wheat flour and all-purpose flour in recipes in the same amount with almost identical results.

Spiced Apple Bread

When shredding your apples, make sure to do it right over the bowl that your batter is in. This will catch all the juices that drip from the apples and give the bread a touch of added moisture and sweetness.

¼ **cup grass-fed butter**

¼ **cup unsweetened applesauce**

½ **cup golden monk fruit sweetener**

½ **cup granulated monk fruit sweetener**

2 large eggs

2 cups cassava flour

1 teaspoon baking soda

½ **teaspoon sea salt**

1½ **teaspoons ground cinnamon**

2 large Fuji apples, peeled and cored

1 Preheat oven to 325°F. Line an 8" × 4" loaf pan with parchment paper.

2 Combine butter, applesauce, and sweeteners in a medium bowl and use a handheld mixer to beat until smooth. Beat in eggs, one at a time.

3 In a separate medium bowl, sift together cassava flour, baking soda, salt, and cinnamon. Fold flour mixture into butter mixture and stir until just combined.

4 Use a cheese grater to shred apples directly over bowl to catch any juice. Stir in shredded apples.

5 Transfer mixture to prepared loaf pan and bake for 1 hour or until a toothpick inserted in the center comes out clean.

6 Allow to cool for 30 minutes before slicing. Once cooled, cut into ten equal-sized slices and serve.

Peanut Butter Banana Smoothie

The banana milk in this recipe adds a touch of sweetness—and a few extra carbohydrates. If you don't have it, you can add a couple extra tablespoons of almond milk until you reach your desired consistency.

1 small peeled ripe banana, frozen

2 tablespoons banana milk

½ cup unsweetened vanilla almond milk

¼ cup creamy no-sugar-added peanut butter

¼ cup frozen chopped spinach

1 tablespoon grass-fed collagen powder

SERVES 1	
Per Serving:	
Calories	574
Fat	37g
Protein	25g
Sodium	174mg
Fiber	8g
Carbohydrates	39g
Net Carbs	31g
Sugar	17g

1 Combine all ingredients in a blender and blend until smooth.

2 Serve immediately.

Chocolate Mint Smoothie

If you don't have fresh mint, you can use ¼ teaspoon of peppermint extract in its place. Keep in mind, if you do, you'll still get a great flavor, but without the health benefits that come with using the fresh stuff.

1 medium peeled banana, frozen and cut in half

½ cup full-fat plain Greek yogurt

1 tablespoon unsweetened cocoa powder

1 tablespoon chopped fresh mint

¼ teaspoon vanilla extract

1 cup unsweetened chocolate almond milk

SERVES 1	
Per Serving:	
Calories	285
Fat	11g
Protein	15g
Sodium	226mg
Fiber	6g
Carbohydrates	38g
Net Carbs	32g
Sugar	20g

1 Combine all ingredients in a blender and blend until smooth.

2 Serve immediately.

Butternut Squash Breakfast Casserole

Per Serving:

Calories	285
Fat	21g
Protein	14g
Sodium	403mg
Fiber	2g
Carbohydrates	10g
Net Carbs	8g
Sugar	3g

Butternut squash doesn't get as much love as pumpkin, but it's a great beta-carotene-rich alternative. Like pumpkin, butternut squash has a slightly sweet flavor that counteracts the paprika just right in this casserole.

2 cups cubed butternut squash

2 tablespoons butter-flavored coconut oil, divided

½ teaspoon sea salt

¼ teaspoon ground black pepper

¼ teaspoon garlic powder

¼ teaspoon paprika

1 teaspoon minced garlic

1 small yellow onion, peeled and diced

1 large green bell pepper, seeded and diced

2 cups chopped kale

8 large eggs

¼ cup full-fat coconut milk

1 tablespoon chopped fresh parsley

1 cup shredded pepper jack cheese

1 Preheat oven to 375°F. Line a baking sheet with parchment paper and spray a 9" × 13" baking dish with coconut oil baking spray.

2 Toss butternut squash with 1 tablespoon coconut oil, salt, pepper, garlic powder, and paprika and arrange in a single layer on baking sheet. Bake for 25 minutes or until tender. Remove from heat.

3 While squash is cooking, heat remaining coconut oil in a medium skillet over medium heat. Add garlic and onion and cook for 1 minute. Add bell pepper and cook for another 5 minutes or until pepper starts to soften. Stir in kale and cook until wilted, about 2 minutes. Remove from heat.

4 Combine eggs and milk in a large mixing bowl and whisk until smooth. Whisk in parsley and cheese. Add pepper mixture and cooked squash and toss to combine. Transfer mixture to prepared baking dish and bake for 30 minutes or until eggs set.

5 Remove from oven and allow to cool slightly before serving.

Butternut Squash Porridge

If you want to add a little texture to this porridge, you can stir in walnuts, almonds, or some no-sugar-added granola after processing it. These keto cycling–friendly toppings will add a nice crunch.

1 large butternut squash, halved and seeded

¼ cup full-fat coconut milk

1 teaspoon ground cinnamon

2 tablespoons golden monk fruit sweetener

1 Preheat oven to 350°F. Line a baking sheet with parchment paper.

2 Place butternut squash, cut side up, on baking sheet and bake for 1 hour or until softened. Allow to cool completely.

3 Remove flesh of squash from skin and transfer to a food processor. Add remaining ingredients and process until smooth, about 1 minute.

4 Remove from food processor and serve immediately.

SERVES 4	
Per Serving:	
Calories	71
Fat	2g
Protein	1g
Sodium	8mg
Fiber	2g
Carbohydrates	19g
Net Carbs	11g
Sugar	3g

Chocolate-Covered Strawberry Smoothie

SERVES 1

Per Serving:

Calories	396
Fat	27g
Protein	13g
Sodium	268mg
Fiber	9g
Carbohydrates	35g
Net Carbs	26g
Sugar	13g

GOING ORGANIC

Did you know that conventionally grown strawberries are one of the "dirtiest" fruits when it comes to pesticides? According to reports by the Environmental Working Group, approximately 99 percent of conventionally grown strawberries contain at least one pesticide; about 30 percent contain at least ten different pesticides; and one sample was found to contain 23 different pesticides. If your budget doesn't allow for you to purchase all organic produce, prioritize strawberries.

Conventional chocolate-covered strawberries are full of added sugars and not really appropriate for breakfast. Enter: this Chocolate-Covered Strawberry Smoothie. It gives you all the great taste of a chocolate-covered strawberry, but it's packed with nutrition, unlike the "real" thing.

¾ cup unsweetened chocolate almond milk

2 tablespoons banana milk

1 tablespoon unsweetened cocoa powder

3 raw Brazil nuts

1 teaspoon melted coconut oil

½ cup frozen strawberries

½ medium peeled banana, frozen

1 tablespoon chocolate MCT oil powder

½ cup frozen chopped spinach

1 tablespoon grass-fed collagen powder

1 Combine all ingredients in a blender and blend until smooth.

2 Serve immediately.

Pumpkin Cinnamon Waffles

Although the waffles come out crisp right off the waffle iron, they may get a little soft as you wait for the others to cook. If this happens, and you want to crisp them up, you can pop them in the toaster for a minute before serving.

3 large eggs, separated

1 cup pumpkin purée

1 cup unsweetened vanilla almond milk

1 cup cassava flour

½ cup paleo flour

1 tablespoon baking powder

1 tablespoon granulated monk fruit sweetener

½ teaspoon sea salt

1 teaspoon ground cinnamon

3 tablespoons grass-fed butter, melted

¼ cup monk fruit–sweetened maple syrup

¼ cup no-sugar-added creamy peanut butter, melted

1 Preheat waffle iron.

2 Place egg yolks and egg whites into two separate medium bowls.

3 Add pumpkin purée and almond milk to egg yolks and stir until smooth. Set aside.

4 In a separate medium bowl, sift together cassava flour, paleo flour, baking powder, sweetener, salt, and cinnamon. Fold flour mixture into pumpkin mixture and stir until just incorporated.

5 Beat egg whites with a handheld mixer until stiff peaks form, about 2 minutes. Fold egg whites into batter. Stir in melted butter.

6 Cook batter in batches, following the instructions from your waffle iron's manufacturer.

7 Serve waffles with monk fruit–sweetened maple syrup and a drizzle of melted peanut butter.

**SERVES 6
(MAKES 6 WAFFLES)**

Per Serving:

Calories	289
Fat	16g
Protein	8g
Sodium	505mg
Fiber	5g
Carbohydrates	30g
Net Carbs	15g
Sugar	2g

THE PURPOSE OF WHIPPED EGG WHITES

Whipped egg whites introduce air into a recipe and help make the finished product lighter and fluffier. There are two stages of whipped egg whites: soft peaks and stiff peaks. As you're beating the eggs, you'll notice peaks start to form. If you lift your beater out of the eggs and the tip of the peak folds over, those are soft peaks. If you lift your beater out of the eggs and they hold their shape, those are stiff peaks.

Butternut Squash Hash

You can make this hash a complete breakfast by combining it with a couple of over-easy eggs, some slices of avocado, and a few dashes of hot sauce.

SERVES 4

Per Serving:

Calories	214
Fat	11g
Protein	7g
Sodium	875mg
Fiber	4g
Carbohydrates	24g
Net Carbs	20g
Sugar	10g

3 cups cubed butternut squash

1 tablespoon olive oil

1 teaspoon sea salt

8 slices no-sugar-added bacon, chopped

1 small yellow onion, peeled and diced

1 large Fuji apple, peeled, cored, and shredded

1 Preheat oven to 425°F. Line a baking sheet with parchment paper.

2 Combine butternut squash, olive oil, and salt in a medium bowl and toss to coat. Spread in an even layer on baking sheet.

3 Roast for 30 minutes or until squash is tender and starts to brown, turning once during cooking. Remove from oven and set aside.

4 Heat a medium skillet over medium-high heat. Once the pan is hot, add bacon and cook for 2 minutes. Stir in onions and cook for an additional 2 minutes. Add apples and cook until softened, about 3 minutes.

5 Add cooked squash to the skillet and stir to combine. Cook for 1 minute or until heated through.

6 Remove from heat and serve.

Pumpkin and Banana Pancakes

Pumpkins and bananas both have natural sugars that give these pancakes the perfect subtle sweetness. Top them with a drizzle of peanut butter and some monk fruit–sweetened maple syrup for a real treat.

⅔ cup pumpkin purée

1 cup mashed peeled overripe banana

6 large eggs

½ teaspoon vanilla extract

¼ cup unsweetened almond milk

¼ cup coconut flour

⅓ cup blanched almond flour

1 teaspoon baking powder

1 teaspoon baking soda

1 teaspoon ground cinnamon

2 tablespoons butter-flavored coconut oil

SERVES 4	
Per Serving:	
Calories	322
Fat	20g
Protein	14g
Sodium	574mg
Fiber	7g
Carbohydrates	24g
Net Carbs	17g
Sugar	9g

1 Combine pumpkin and banana in a medium bowl and beat with a handheld mixer until smooth. Add eggs, vanilla extract, and almond milk and beat until incorporated.

2 In a separate medium bowl, combine remaining ingredients, except coconut oil, and mix until incorporated.

3 Add dry ingredients to pumpkin mixture and stir until just combined.

4 Heat coconut oil in a large skillet or on a griddle over medium heat. Use a ¼ cup measure to scoop batter into hot skillet or on griddle. Cook until bubbles form, about 4 minutes, flip, and then cook for an additional 4 minutes or until golden brown.

5 Remove pancakes from heat and repeat with remaining batter. Serve immediately.

Blueberry Banana Yogurt

SERVES 1	
Per Serving:	
Calories	143
Fat	5g
Protein	6g
Sodium	91mg
Fiber	1g
Carbohydrates	19g
Net Carbs	18g
Sugar	11g

This homemade Blueberry Banana Yogurt is a lower-carb, added sugar–free version of the flavored yogurts you can buy in stores. It will satisfy your sweet tooth without drastic spikes in your blood sugar. You can stir in some nuts or collagen powder for extra protein.

1 (5.3-ounce) container plain full-fat yogurt
½ teaspoon vanilla extract
2 tablespoons mashed peeled ripe banana
¼ cup frozen wild blueberries, thawed
2 teaspoons stevia-sweetened maple syrup

1 Combine all ingredients in a small bowl and stir until smooth.

2 Serve immediately.

Triple Berry Overnight Oats

SERVES 1	
Per Serving:	
Calories	347
Fat	10g
Protein	12g
Sodium	162mg
Fiber	10g
Carbohydrates	55g
Net Carbs	45g
Sugar	18g

As the frozen berries sit in the oat mixture in the refrigerator overnight, they begin to thaw and release their juices. This process adds a nice, natural berry flavor to the oatmeal when you stir it.

½ cup unsweetened vanilla almond milk
½ cup gluten-free oats
½ cup full-fat plain yogurt
½ teaspoon vanilla extract
1 teaspoon chia seeds
½ small peeled overripe banana, mashed
⅓ cup frozen mixed berries

1 Combine all ingredients in a sealable jar and stir to mix.

2 Cover and refrigerate overnight, or at least 6 hours. Serve cold.

Chocolate Chip Banana Bread

This Chocolate Chip Banana Bread has only a touch of added sweetener. It gets most of its sweetness from the bananas, which have a low glycemic index even when they're really ripe.

4 large eggs

3 large overripe bananas, peeled and mashed

2 teaspoons vanilla extract

¼ cup butter-flavored coconut oil, melted

2 tablespoons golden monk fruit sweetener

2¼ cups paleo flour

1 teaspoon baking soda

½ teaspoon baking powder

1 teaspoon ground cinnamon

¼ teaspoon sea salt

½ cup stevia-sweetened chocolate chips

SERVES 10	
Per Serving:	
Calories	271
Fat	15g
Protein	7g
Sodium	231mg
Fiber	5g
Carbohydrates	31g
Net Carbs	23g
Sugar	6g

1 Preheat oven to 325°F. Line an 8" × 4" loaf pan with parchment paper.

2 Combine eggs, bananas, vanilla, coconut oil, and monk fruit sweetener in a medium bowl and whisk together until smooth. Set aside.

3 Combine remaining ingredients, except chocolate chips, in a separate medium bowl. Fold dry ingredients into wet ingredients and stir until just incorporated. Stir in chocolate chips.

4 Transfer batter to prepared loaf pan and bake for 1 hour or until a toothpick inserted in the center comes out clean.

5 Allow to cool and then remove from pan, slice, and serve.

Ginger Pumpkin Bread

YOUR OWN PUMPKIN PIE SPICE BLEND

If you don't have pre-made pumpkin pie spice on hand, you can make your own by combining 3 teaspoons ground cinnamon, ¾ teaspoon ground nutmeg, ¾ teaspoon ground ginger, and ⅛ teaspoon ground cloves. Use what you need and store the rest in an airtight container for up to 6 months in your spice cabinet until you're ready to use it.

The spicy kick of the ginger in this bread gives a nice contrast to its sweetness. If you're not a ginger lover, you can simply omit it and throw in a little extra pumpkin pie spice to balance it out.

1½ cups blanched almond flour

½ teaspoon sea salt

¾ teaspoon baking soda

3 teaspoons pumpkin pie spice

¼ teaspoon ground ginger

4 large eggs

¾ cup pumpkin purée

¼ cup monk fruit–sweetened maple syrup

1 teaspoon vanilla extract

1 Preheat oven to 350°F. Coat an 8.5" × 4.5" loaf pan with coconut oil baking spray.

2 Combine almond flour, salt, baking soda, pumpkin pie spice, and ginger in a medium mixing bowl. Mix well.

3 In a separate medium bowl, combine remaining ingredients and whisk until smooth. Fold wet ingredients into dry ingredients and stir until just incorporated.

4 Pour mixture into prepared loaf pan and spread evenly. Bake for 40 minutes or until a toothpick inserted in the center comes out clean.

5 Allow to cool, then cut into ten equal-sized slices and serve.

Pumpkin Parfait

The riper the banana you use for this recipe, the better! Bananas get sweeter as they ripen, and the natural sugar will counteract the tartness of the plain yogurt.

1 cup full-fat plain yogurt

8 ounces cream cheese, softened

1 tablespoon fresh orange juice

1 (14-ounce) can pumpkin purée

¼ cup monk fruit–sweetened maple syrup

2 teaspoons ground cinnamon

½ cup mashed peeled ripe banana

¼ cup crushed walnuts

1 Combine yogurt, cream cheese, and orange juice in a medium bowl and beat with a handheld mixer until smooth. Set aside.

2 In a separate medium bowl, combine pumpkin purée, maple syrup, and cinnamon and stir until smooth.

3 Divide yogurt mixture in half and fold half into pumpkin mixture, stirring just enough to combine.

4 Divide pumpkin mixture evenly among four glass bowls. Scoop equal amounts of mashed banana on top, then top with equal amounts of yogurt mixture.

5 Refrigerate for 3 hours.

6 Sprinkle crushed walnuts on top before serving.

SERVES 4

Per Serving:

Calories	361
Fat	27g
Protein	8g
Sodium	242mg
Fiber	6g
Carbohydrates	28g
Net Carbs	6g
Sugar	13g

THE SUGAR IN YOGURT

Flavored yogurts and those with fruit on the bottom contain just about 26 grams of sugar, which is close to the amount in a can of soda! Some of this sugar is naturally occurring, but about 14 grams are added—and those are the grams you want to avoid. Steer clear of any flavored yogurts or yogurts with added fruit or granola and opt for plain, full-fat varieties.

Apple Cinnamon Waffles

No matter what waffle iron you're using, a good way to tell if your waffles are almost done is by the steam. While they're cooking, waffles will steam a lot. As they get close to being done, the steam will dissipate and you can open the iron and check them.

1½ cups cassava flour

2 tablespoons granulated monk fruit sweetener

1 teaspoon baking powder

½ teaspoon baking soda

1 teaspoon ground cinnamon

½ teaspoon ground nutmeg

½ teaspoon sea salt

2 large eggs

1¼ cups unsweetened vanilla almond milk

⅔ cup unsweetened applesauce

2 tablespoons golden monk fruit sweetener

½ cup grass-fed butter, melted

1 teaspoon vanilla extract

2 medium Fuji apples, cored, shredded, and squeezed dry

1 Preheat waffle iron.

2 Sift together cassava flour, granulated monk fruit sweetener, baking powder, baking soda, cinnamon, nutmeg, and salt in a medium mixing bowl.

3 In a separate medium bowl, lightly whisk eggs and then add almond milk, applesauce, golden monk fruit sweetener, melted butter, and vanilla extract. Stir until combined.

4 Fold wet ingredients into dry ingredients and mix until just combined. Stir apples into batter.

5 Add batter to preheated waffle iron in batches and cook according to the manufacturer's instructions.

6 Remove waffles from heat and serve immediately.

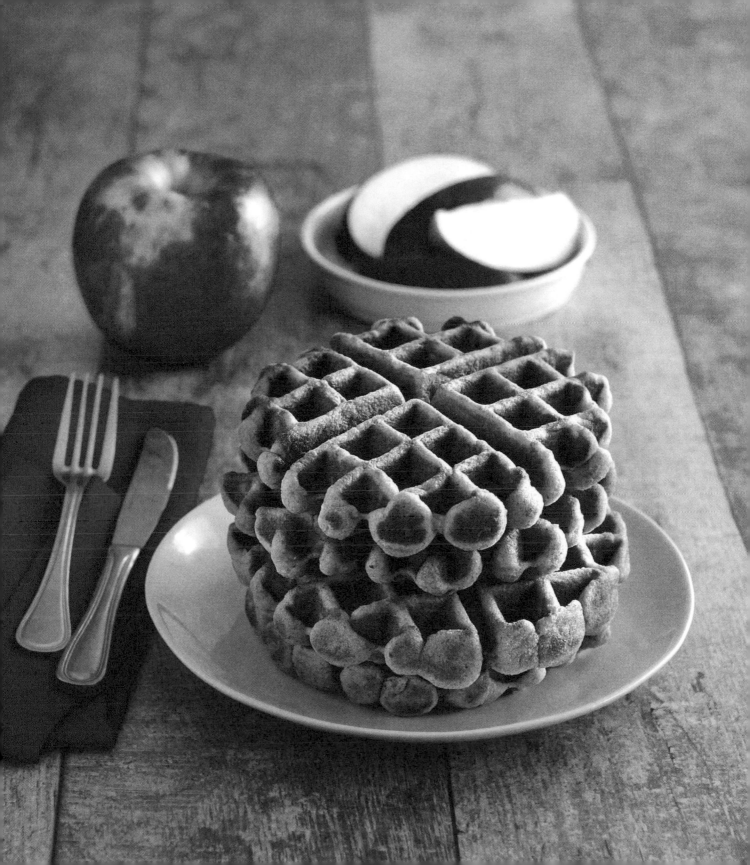

Spiced Sweet Potato Pancakes

These Spiced Sweet Potato Pancakes combine all of the best flavors of cool weather into one easy-to-prepare breakfast. They hit the spot anytime of the year!

SERVES 6	
Per Serving:	
Calories	283
Fat	14g
Protein	6g
Sodium	625mg
Fiber	4g
Carbohydrates	40g
Net Carbs	30g
Sugar	3g

MAKING YOUR OWN PURÉE

Sweet potato purée is available canned right where you'd find the pumpkin purée, but if you prefer, you can make your own by roasting whole sweet potatoes at 425°F for 45 minutes or until they're soft, allowing them to cool, peeling off the skin, and transferring the flesh into a food processor and processing until smooth. If you make more than you need, you can freeze the purée in small batches for up to 6 months and use them as needed.

1½ cups unsweetened vanilla almond milk

1 cup sweet potato purée

1 large egg

2 tablespoons grass-fed butter, melted

1 cup paleo flour

1 cup cassava flour

3 tablespoons golden monk fruit sweetener

2 teaspoons baking powder

1 teaspoon baking soda

1 teaspoon ground cinnamon

½ teaspoon ground ginger

¼ teaspoon ground cloves

½ teaspoon sea salt

2 tablespoons butter-flavored coconut oil

1 Combine almond milk, sweet potato, egg, and butter in a medium bowl and whisk until smooth.

2 In a separate medium bowl, sift together paleo flour, cassava flour, monk fruit sweetener, baking powder, baking soda, cinnamon, ginger, cloves, and salt.

3 Fold flour mixture into sweet potato mixture and stir just enough to combine.

4 Heat coconut oil in a large skillet or on a griddle over medium heat. Using a ¼ cup measure, scoop batter and pour into hot skillet or on griddle.

5 Cook until bubbles start to form, about 3 minutes, flip, and then cook for another 3 minutes or until golden brown.

6 Remove from heat and serve warm.

CHAPTER 11

Carb-Day Lunch

Apple and Pork Burgers

Gala apples have a mildly sweet flavor that complements the saltiness of the ground pork nicely. If you want to kick up the apple flavor, serve these with a dollop of unsweetened applesauce on top.

SERVES 6	
Per Serving:	
Calories	455
Fat	31g
Protein	34g
Sodium	365mg
Fiber	1g
Carbohydrates	9g
Net Carbs	8g
Sugar	6g

MAKING YOUR OWN TERIYAKI SAUCE

Even on your higher-carb days, it's best to make your own teriyaki sauce so you can control the ingredient list. Combine ½ cup coconut aminos, ¼ cup orange juice, 3 tablespoons raw honey, 2 teaspoons grated ginger, 2 teaspoons minced garlic, and ⅛ teaspoon red pepper flakes in a medium saucepan over medium heat, stirring occasionally. While sauce is cooking, stir 2 teaspoons arrowroot powder with 2 tablespoons cold water in a small bowl. Add to sauce and simmer until thickened, about 5 minutes.

1½ pounds ground pork

1 small Gala apple, peeled, cored, and minced

1 small sweet onion, peeled and minced

2 teaspoons minced garlic

¼ cup coarse almond meal

¼ cup homemade teriyaki sauce

1 large egg

6 slices Swiss cheese

1 Preheat outdoor grill to medium-high heat.

2 Combine all ingredients except Swiss cheese in a medium bowl and mix until incorporated. Form into six equal-sized patties.

3 Transfer burgers to hot grill and cook for 5 minutes, flip, and then cook for another 5 minutes or until pork is no longer pink.

4 Place a slice of Swiss cheese on top of each burger and cook for 1 more minute until cheese melts.

5 Remove from heat and serve.

Thyme Chicken Soup

The brown rice in this recipe provides important macronutrients for your high-carb days. If you want to enjoy this dish on your lower-carb days, omit the rice and cut down the amount of carrots, if you need to.

1 whole rotisserie chicken

12 cups chicken bone broth

¼ cup grass-fed butter

1 teaspoon minced garlic

2 large yellow onions, peeled and chopped

3 large carrots, peeled and cut into half-rounds

2 medium stalks celery, cut into half-moons

1 teaspoon dried thyme

1 cup cooked long-grain sprouted brown rice

1 Separate chicken meat from bones and set meat aside in a medium bowl. Transfer bones and skin to a large stockpot.

2 Pour chicken broth over bones and bring to a simmer over medium-high heat. Once broth starts to simmer, reduce heat to low and cover. Simmer for 1 hour.

3 Pour broth through a strainer into a large bowl. Discard bones and set broth aside.

4 Return stockpot to stove at medium heat and add butter. When butter is hot, add garlic and onions and cook for 1 minute. Add carrots and celery and continue cooking until soft, about 7 minutes.

5 Pour broth back into pot. Stir in thyme and chicken.

6 Allow to simmer, then reduce heat to low. Simmer for 1 hour. Stir in rice and cook for 5 minutes or until heated through.

7 Allow to cool slightly before serving.

SERVES 6

Per Serving:

Calories	303
Fat	10g
Protein	36g
Sodium	821mg
Fiber	3g
Carbohydrates	17g
Net Carbs	14g
Sugar	4g

LONG GRAIN VERSUS SHORT GRAIN

The grain of rice refers to the grain's length-to-width ratio. Long-grain rice is long and thin, while short-grain rice is wider than it is long. Long-grain rice is also less starchy (and slightly lower in carbohydrates), while short-grain rice contains a lot of starch and, because of this, tends to stick together. When using long-grain rice, you'll get distinct pieces of rice, but short-grain will clump together. You can use either one, but keep in mind that it may change the texture of the recipe.

Loaded Baked "Potato" Soup

This Loaded Baked "Potato" Soup gives you the familiar comfort of the real thing, but with significantly fewer carbs. The base is made from cauliflower, so you can still enjoy some potatoes while staying in ketosis.

8 slices no-sugar-added bacon, roughly chopped

2 teaspoons minced garlic

1 cup chopped leeks

¾ cup chopped celery

4 cups chicken bone broth

8 cups chopped cauliflower florets

¾ teaspoon sea salt

¼ teaspoon ground black pepper

¾ cup grass-fed half-and-half

¼ cup sour cream

2 medium baked russet potatoes, skins removed and roughly chopped

¾ cup shredded Cheddar cheese

2 tablespoons chopped fresh chives

1 Heat a large stockpot over medium heat. Add bacon and cook until crisp, about 7 minutes. Remove bacon from pan and transfer to a paper towel–lined plate.

2 Reserve 2 tablespoons of bacon grease and discard the rest.

3 Add garlic and leeks to the pan and cook for 1 minute. Add celery and cook until tender, but still a little crisp, about 5 minutes.

4 Pour broth into pot and stir in cauliflower, salt, and pepper. Increase heat to high and bring to a boil. Once mixture starts boiling, reduce to low and simmer until cauliflower softens, about 10 minutes.

5 Use an immersion blender to purée soup to desired consistency. Stir in half-and-half and sour cream until smooth.

6 Stir in potatoes. Remove from heat and top with Cheddar cheese, chives, and bacon before serving.

Curried Chicken Salad

This Curried Chicken Salad is even better after it sits in the refrigerator for 24 hours and the flavors have had a chance to meld together. Prepare it in advance or as part of a meal prep routine for the greatest flavor payoff.

2 cups cooked diced chicken

1 medium stalk celery, finely diced

1 large green apple, cored and finely diced

⅓ cup green grapes, cut in half

¼ cup crushed walnuts

½ cup keto-friendly mayonnaise

¼ teaspoon sea salt

¼ teaspoon ground black pepper

¼ teaspoon curry powder

SERVES 4	
Per Serving:	
Calories	379
Fat	32g
Protein	14g
Sodium	467mg
Fiber	2g
Carbohydrates	13g
Net Carbs	11g
Sugar	8g

1 Combine all ingredients in a large bowl and stir until fully incorporated.

2 Chill for at least 1 hour before serving.

Beet and Goat Cheese Mason Jar Salad

This Beet and Goat Cheese Mason Jar Salad calls for spiralized beets, but if you don't have a spiralizer, don't worry! You can get the same great flavor just by roughly chopping your beets and adding them to your salad that way.

¼ cup Tessemae's Organic Lemon Garlic Dressing & Marinade

½ cup cooked cubed chicken

1 large beet, peeled and spiralized

½ cup crumbled goat cheese

½ cup crushed raw walnuts

2 cups arugula

SERVES 2	
Per Serving:	
Calories	528
Fat	48g
Protein	18g
Sodium	444mg
Fiber	5g
Carbohydrates	13g
Net Carbs	8g
Sugar	6g

1 Place 2 tablespoons of dressing into the bottom of each of two 32-ounce Mason jars. Layer each jar with ¼ cup chicken, ½ spiralized beet, ¼ cup goat cheese, ¼ cup walnuts, and 1 cup arugula.

2 Cover and store in the refrigerator for up to 1 week. When ready to eat, shake vigorously before serving.

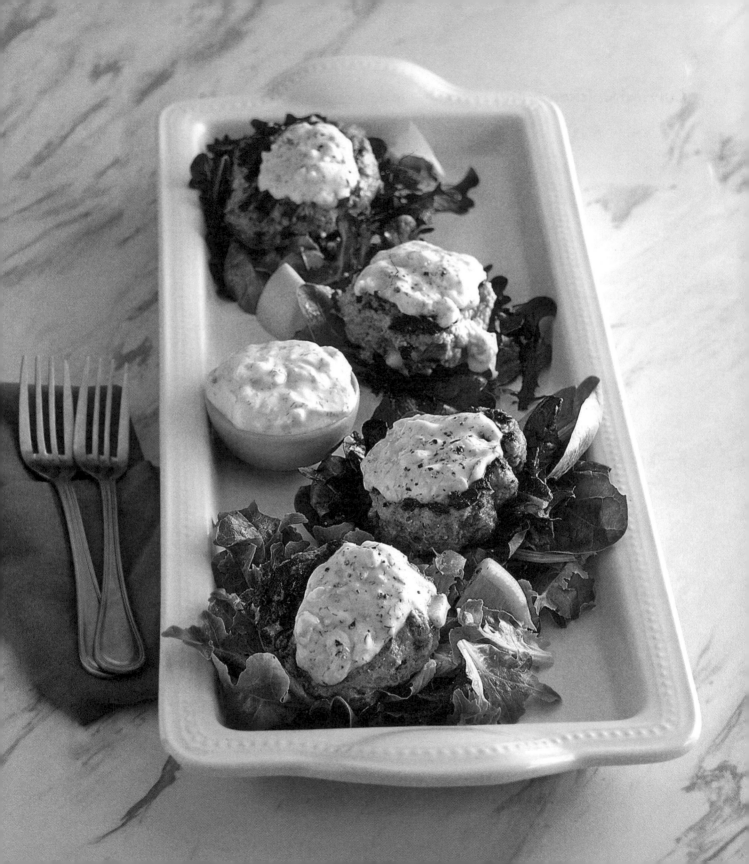

Sun-Dried Tomato and Feta Chicken Burgers with Cucumber Dill Sauce

These burgers bring the best Greek flavors together in one per-fectly balanced dish for a high-carb day. Serve them with a side of Herb-Roasted Turnips (see recipe in Chapter 5) to make your meal really hearty.

SERVES 6	
Per Serving:	
Calories	444
Fat	36g
Protein	27g
Sodium	597mg
Fiber	2g
Carbohydrates	7g
Net Carbs	5g
Sugar	3g

Burgers

1 tablespoon avocado oil

1½ pounds ground chicken

½ cup coarse almond meal

1 large egg

1 tablespoon lemon juice

¼ cup chopped sun-dried tomatoes

1½ tablespoons chopped fresh basil

1 teaspoon dried oregano

½ teaspoon sea salt

½ teaspoon ground black pepper

⅓ cup crumbled feta cheese

Cucumber Dill Sauce

1 small cucumber, peeled, seeded, and minced

½ cup full-fat plain Greek yogurt

½ cup keto-friendly mayonnaise

¼ teaspoon white vinegar

⅛ teaspoon lemon juice

½ teaspoon minced garlic

2 tablespoons crumbled feta cheese

½ teaspoon dried chives

½ teaspoon dried dill

⅛ teaspoon dried oregano

¼ teaspoon sea salt

¼ teaspoon ground black pepper

1 **For Burgers:** Preheat outdoor grill to medium-high heat. Brush oil on grill grate. Combine all ingredients in a medium bowl and mix with your hands until incorporated. Form mixture into six patties. Cook on preheated grill for 5 minutes, flip, and then cook for another 5 minutes or until chicken is no longer pink and juices run clear.

2 **For Cucumber Dill Sauce:** While burgers are cooking, com-bine all ingredients for sauce in a separate medium mixing bowl. Whisk to combine.

3 Remove burgers from grill and top each with 2½ tablespoons dill sauce. Serve immediately.

Mason Jar Burrito Bowls

You can enjoy all the flavors of a burrito without the processed tortilla shells and toppings. This recipe is a perfect grab-and-go lunch option because you can prepare a few in advance and take them with you when you need them.

4 tablespoons Tessemae's Organic Habanero Ranch Dressing

2 tablespoons minced seeded green bell pepper

2 tablespoons chopped black olives

1 cup cooked black beans

½ cup cooked taco meat

2 tablespoons shredded Cheddar cheese

1 cup cooked sprouted brown rice

2 cups chopped romaine lettuce

1 Scoop 2 tablespoons of dressing into each of two 32-ounce wide-mouthed Mason jars.

2 Layer 1 tablespoon bell peppers, 1 tablespoon olives, ½ cup black beans, ¼ cup taco meat, 1 tablespoon shredded Cheddar cheese, ½ cup brown rice, and 1 cup romaine lettuce in each jar.

3 Cover and store in the refrigerator until ready to eat, up to 1 week. Shake vigorously before serving.

Spinach, Feta, and Beet Mason Jar Salad

The earthy flavor of beets is offset with the salty creaminess of feta cheese in this easy-to-put-together salad. The classic spinach-feta combination complements the beets nicely.

4 tablespoons Tessemae's Organic Lemon Garlic Dressing & Marinade

1 cup peeled, chopped cooked beets

¼ cup shredded peeled carrots

2 tablespoons minced peeled red onion

½ cup shredded cooked chicken

½ cup crumbled feta cheese

¼ cup crushed walnuts

2 cups baby spinach

SERVES 2	
Per Serving:	
Calories	451
Fat	36g
Protein	21g
Sodium	736mg
Fiber	5g
Carbohydrates	11g
Net Carbs	6g
Sugar	4g

1 Scoop 2 tablespoons dressing into the bottom of two 32-ounce widemouthed Mason jars.

2 Layer ½ cup beets, 2 tablespoons carrots, 1 tablespoon onion, ¼ cup chicken, ¼ cup feta cheese, 2 tablespoons walnuts, and 1 cup spinach in each jar.

3 Cover and refrigerate until ready to eat, up to 1 week. Shake vigorously before serving.

Beef, Brown Rice, and Kale Bowls

These bowls contain different types of complex carbohydrates (carrots and rice) to help you maximize your intake of important vitamins and minerals on your high-carb day. You can add some healthy fats by topping with a sliced avocado or some keto-friendly ranch dressing.

SERVES 4	
Per Serving:	
Calories	255
Fat	13g
Protein	17g
Sodium	914mg
Fiber	2g
Carbohydrates	17g
Net Carbs	15g
Sugar	4g

1 cup sprouted brown rice

2 cups chicken bone broth

2 tablespoons grass-fed butter

1 teaspoon minced garlic

¼ cup chopped peeled yellow onion

½ cup chopped celery

½ cup shredded peeled carrots

½ pound 85/15 ground beef

½ cup sliced mushrooms

2 cups chopped kale

1 teaspoon sea salt

3 tablespoons coconut aminos

1 Combine brown rice and broth in a medium saucepan over high heat. Bring to a boil, cover, and reduce heat to low. Simmer until liquid has been absorbed and rice is tender and fluffy, about 45 minutes. Remove from heat.

2 Add butter to a large saucepan over medium heat. Add garlic and onion and cook for 1 minute. Stir in celery and carrot and cook until they start to soften, about 5 minutes. Add ground beef and cook for 5 minutes, stirring frequently. Stir in mushrooms and cook for another 3 minutes or until beef is no longer pink.

3 Add brown rice and kale and stir to combine. Cook until kale wilts, about 2 minutes. Stir in salt and coconut aminos.

4 Remove from heat and serve.

Broccoli Slaw and Wild Rice Mason Jar Salad

This recipe uses the Fresh Broccoli Slaw from Chapter 5. The slaw adds a sweet, creamy crunchiness to the salad that blends well with the savory wild rice.

2 tablespoons Tessemae's Organic Creamy Ranch Dressing

½ cup chopped seeded red bell pepper

½ cup shredded peeled carrots

½ cup canned wild Atlantic salmon

1 cup cooked wild rice

2 tablespoons slivered almonds

¼ cup chopped avocado

1 cup Fresh Broccoli Slaw

1 Scoop 1 tablespoon of dressing into each of two 32-ounce wide-mouthed Mason jars.

2 Layer ¼ cup bell peppers, ¼ cup carrots, ¼ cup salmon, ½ cup rice, 1 tablespoon almonds, 2 tablespoons avocado, and ½ cup Fresh Broccoli Slaw in each jar.

3 Cover and refrigerate until ready to eat, up to 1 week. Shake vigorously before serving.

SERVES 2	
Per Serving:	
Calories	368
Fat	17g
Protein	20g
Sodium	352mg
Fiber	5g
Carbohydrates	28g
Net Carbs	23g
Sugar	4g

JARRED SALADS

You can use any kind of Mason jars you want to make Mason jar salads, but the best option is one that's at least 32 ounces and has a wide mouth. If you choose this combo, it will be easier to fit everything you need into it and get everything out when it's time to eat.

Black Bean and Avocado Mason Jar Salad

Per Serving:

Calories	573
Fat	21g
Protein	33g
Sodium	629mg
Fiber	11g
Carbohydrates	46g
Net Carbs	35g
Sugar	3g

FILL UP ON FIBER

Black beans are one of the most fiber-rich foods around. A single cup of the legumes contains about 15 grams of fiber, roughly half of the amount you need for the entire day. Including beans in your meals on your high-carb days will slow down your digestion and the absorption of the other carbohydrates in your meal. This prevents the spikes in blood sugar that are associated with insulin resistance and weight gain.

If you want to spice this salad up a bit, you can add a few splashes of hot sauce in with the ranch dressing when you're layering your jars. You'll get some heat once you mix it all together.

4 tablespoons Tessemae's Organic Avocado Ranch Dressing

2 tablespoons minced peeled red onion

1 cup cooked black beans

1 cup canned shredded chicken

1 cup cooked sprouted quinoa

2 tablespoons shredded Cheddar cheese

¼ cup chopped avocado

¼ cup chopped cilantro

2 cups chopped romaine lettuce

1 Scoop 2 tablespoons of dressing into the bottom of two 32-ounce widemouthed Mason jars.

2 Layer 1 tablespoon onion, ½ cup black beans, ½ cup chicken, ½ cup quinoa, 1 tablespoon Cheddar cheese, 2 tablespoons avocado, 2 tablespoons cilantro, and 1 cup lettuce in each jar.

3 Cover and store in the refrigerator until ready to eat, up to 1 week. Shake vigorously before serving.

Mulligatawny Soup

Mulligatawny soup is known for its spice. In keeping with tradition, this Mulligatawny Soup packs a little heat. If you want to dial it back, you can leave out the cayenne pepper.

¼ cup grass-fed butter

½ cup chopped peeled yellow onion

3 medium stalks celery, diced

2 medium carrots, peeled and diced

1 tablespoon arrowroot powder

1 tablespoon curry powder

1 teaspoon garam masala

4 cups chicken bone broth

½ Fuji apple, cored and diced

¼ cup long-grain sprouted brown rice

1 cup shredded cooked chicken

1 teaspoon sea salt

½ teaspoon ground black pepper

¼ teaspoon cayenne pepper

⅛ teaspoon dried thyme

½ cup full-fat coconut milk

1 cup chopped fresh spinach

SERVES 6	
Per Serving:	
Calories	244
Fat	15g
Protein	12g
Sodium	621mg
Fiber	3g
Carbohydrates	15g
Net Carbs	12g
Sugar	4g

1 Heat butter in a large stockpot over medium heat. Add onion and cook for 2 minutes. Add celery and carrots and cook until they start to soften, about 5 minutes. Stir in arrowroot powder, curry powder, and garam masala and cook for another 3 minutes.

2 Pour in chicken broth and increase heat to high. Bring to a boil and then reduce heat to low and simmer for 1 hour.

3 Add apple, rice, chicken, salt, black pepper, cayenne pepper, and thyme and simmer for 45 minutes or until rice is tender.

4 Remove 1 cup of soup mixture from pot and blend in a high-powered blender. Stir puréed soup back into pot, along with coconut milk and spinach.

5 Cook until spinach wilts, about 2 minutes.

6 Remove from heat and serve warm.

Quinoa Pad Thai

This version of Pad Thai replaces rice noodles with quinoa, a more complex carbohydrate that is lower in total carbohydrates and higher in fiber and contains almost three times as much protein.

RINSING YOUR QUINOA

Quinoa has a natural coating, called *saponin*, on it. The saponin can make the quinoa taste bitter or soapy, and it's often the reason people think they don't like quinoa. If your quinoa isn't pre-rinsed, you can remove the saponin by rinsing quinoa in a fine-mesh strainer under cold running water for 2 minutes before using it in your recipes.

Pad Thai

2 cups chicken bone broth

1 cup sprouted quinoa

1 tablespoon avocado oil

½ pound boneless, skinless chicken thighs, cubed

½ cup shredded green cabbage

¼ cup shredded broccoli stems

2 large carrots, peeled and julienned

3 green onions, chopped

2 large eggs

1 teaspoon sesame oil

Peanut Sauce

¼ cup no-sugar-added crunchy peanut butter

¼ cup coconut aminos

2 tablespoons rice vinegar

1 tablespoon red chili paste

1 tablespoon sriracha

1 teaspoon minced garlic

1 teaspoon ground ginger

¼ teaspoon crushed red pepper

1 teaspoon sesame oil

1 teaspoon lime juice

2 tablespoons full-fat coconut milk

¼ cup chopped salted peanuts

1 **For Pad Thai:** Combine chicken broth and quinoa in a medium saucepan and stir. Bring to a boil over high heat. Reduce heat to low, cover, and simmer for 15 minutes or until water is absorbed and quinoa is tender. Set aside. Heat oil in a large skillet over medium-high heat. Add chicken and cook until no longer pink, about 7 minutes. Remove chicken from skillet. Add cabbage, broccoli, carrots, and green onions to skillet. Cook for 3 minutes. Combine eggs and sesame oil in a medium bowl and whisk until smooth. Pour eggs in with vegetables and scramble for 2 minutes.

2 **For Peanut Sauce:** Whisk together all Peanut Sauce ingredients in a medium bowl until smooth. Pour sauce over cooked vegetables and toss to coat. Add cooked chicken and quinoa to pan and toss again to coat with sauce. Remove from heat and serve warm.

Creamy Sweet Potato Soup

Cinnamon and nutmeg lend a subtle sweetness to this soup, while ginger and red pepper counteract it with a spicy kick.

3 large sweet potatoes, peeled and cubed

¼ cup chopped peeled white onion

5 cups chicken bone broth

¼ cup golden monk fruit sweetener

½ teaspoon sea salt

¼ teaspoon ground cinnamon

¼ teaspoon ground nutmeg

¹⁄₁₆ teaspoon ground ginger

¼ teaspoon ground black pepper

¹⁄₁₆ teaspoon crushed red pepper

⅓ cup full-fat coconut milk

SERVES 6	
Per Serving:	
Calories	136
Fat	3g
Protein	8g
Sodium	406mg
Fiber	3g
Carbohydrates	28g
Net Carbs	17g
Sugar	6g

1 Combine sweet potatoes, onion, and broth in a large stockpot over medium heat. Cook until sweet potatoes are tender, about 30 minutes.

2 Using an immersion blender, purée soup until smooth.

3 Stir in remaining ingredients. Serve warm.

Beef and Quinoa Mason Jar Salad

Mason jar salads are a great way to take lunch with you on the go. They're easy to put together, portable, and filling.

4 tablespoons Tessemae's Organic Creamy Ranch Dressing

2 tablespoons minced seeded green bell pepper

½ cup cooked 85/15 ground beef

2 tablespoons shredded Cheddar cheese

1 cup cooked sprouted quinoa

2 cups baby kale

SERVES 2	
Per Serving:	
Calories	398
Fat	19g
Protein	13g
Sodium	291mg
Fiber	3g
Carbohydrates	23g
Net Carbs	20g
Sugar	2g

1 Scoop 2 tablespoons of dressing into the bottom of each of two 32-ounce widemouthed Mason jars.

2 Layer each jar with 1 tablespoon green pepper, ¼ cup ground beef, 1 tablespoon Cheddar cheese, ½ cup quinoa, and 1 cup baby kale.

3 Cover and store in the refrigerator until ready to eat, up to 1 week. Shake vigorously before serving.

Mediterranean Quinoa Salad

HOMEMADE CHICKEN SEASONING

To make your own chicken seasoning, combine 2 tablespoons coarse black pepper, 2 tablespoons garlic powder, 2 tablespoons sea salt, 2 tablespoons paprika, 1 tablespoon onion powder, 1 tablespoon ground coriander, 1 tablespoon dried dill, and 1 tablespoon crushed red pepper. Use what you need and store the rest in an airtight container for up to 6 months in your spice cabinet.

You can enjoy this Mediterranean Quinoa Salad warm after cooking, or refrigerate it for a couple of hours if you prefer to eat it chilled. Either way, it's a delicious way to get those complex carbohydrates in.

1 cup chicken bone broth

½ cup sprouted quinoa

3 tablespoons olive oil, divided

12 ounces boneless, skinless chicken breasts, cubed

1 tablespoon chicken seasoning

2 tablespoons fresh lemon juice

2 teaspoons red wine vinegar

¼ teaspoon sea salt

¼ teaspoon Greek oregano

1 small red onion, peeled and minced

1 small red bell pepper, seeded and diced

1 small cucumber, diced

¼ cup chopped pitted Kalamata olives

¼ cup chopped sun-dried tomatoes

¼ cup crumbled feta cheese

2 tablespoons chopped fresh parsley

1 tablespoon dried chives

1 Combine chicken broth and quinoa in a medium saucepan and stir. Bring to a boil over high heat. Reduce heat to low, cover, and simmer for 15 minutes or until water is absorbed and quinoa is tender. Set aside.

2 Heat 1 tablespoon olive oil in a medium skillet over medium heat. Add chicken and cook for 2 minutes, stirring occasionally. Sprinkle chicken seasoning on top of chicken and stir to combine. Continue cooking until chicken is no longer pink, about 5 minutes. Remove from heat and allow to cool slightly.

3 Combine remaining olive oil, lemon juice, red wine vinegar, salt, and oregano in a large bowl and whisk to incorporate.

4 Add remaining ingredients, along with cooked quinoa and cooked chicken, to bowl and toss to coat.

5 Serve.

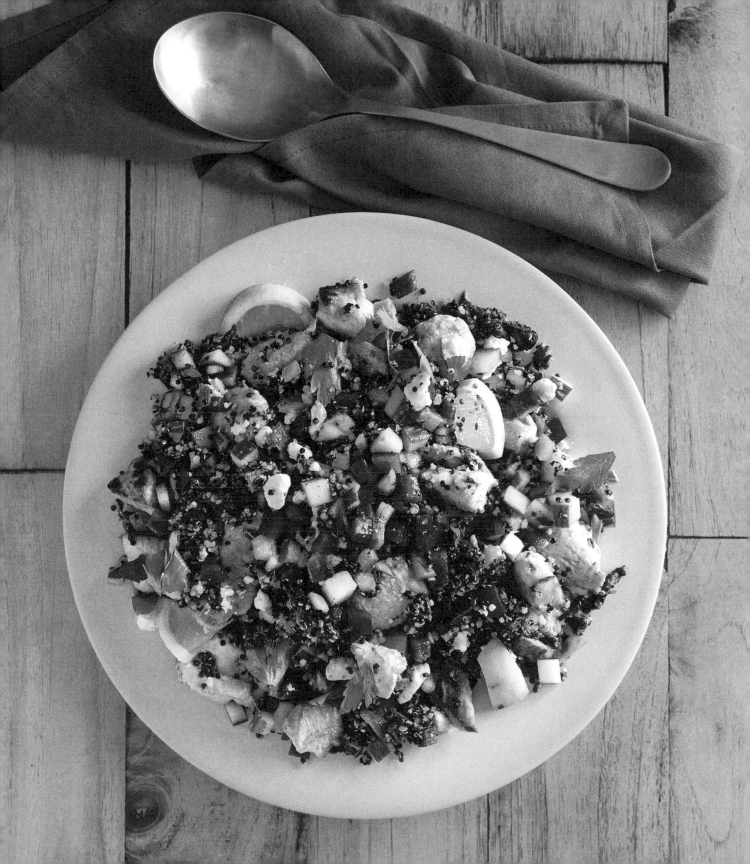

Kale Salad with Quinoa and Avocado

SERVES 4

Per Serving:

Calories	380
Fat	26g
Protein	11g
Sodium	361mg
Fiber	7g
Carbohydrates	29g
Net Carbs	22g
Sugar	4g

EASY LEMON GARLIC DRESSING

If you don't have any keto-friendly dressings on hand, you can make an easy lemon garlic dressing by whisking together ¼ cup olive oil, 2 tablespoons lemon juice, 2 tablespoons Dijon mustard, 1 teaspoon minced garlic, ½ teaspoon sea salt, and ¼ teaspoon ground black pepper.

Massaging the kale for a few minutes with lemon helps break down the kale, softening it so that it's easier to chew and digest. If you prefer (and want to make this a warm salad), you can steam the kale for about a minute before adding it to the bowl.

1⅓ cups chicken bone broth

⅔ cup sprouted quinoa

4 cups chopped kale

⅓ cup Tessemae's Organic Lemon Garlic Dressing & Marinade

⅛ teaspoon sea salt

1 large avocado, peeled, pitted, and chopped

1 large cucumber, chopped

½ cup chopped grape tomatoes

3 tablespoons minced peeled red onion

¼ cup crumbled feta cheese

2 tablespoons pine nuts

1 Combine chicken broth and quinoa in a medium saucepan and stir. Bring to a boil over high heat. Reduce heat to low, cover, and simmer for 15 minutes or until water is absorbed and quinoa is tender. Set aside.

2 While quinoa cooks, add kale to a large bowl, pour dressing on top and sprinkle with salt. Massage dressing into kale for 2 to 3 minutes or until kale starts to wilt.

3 Add remaining ingredients, including cooked quinoa, and toss to coat.

4 Serve.

Spicy Black Bean Soup

After cooking this soup, you can let it cool and then divide it into eight equal portions. Eat what you want on your high-carb day and then freeze the rest for up to 6 months. That way, you'll have a freezer stocked full of future lunches.

1 tablespoon olive oil

1 medium white onion, peeled and chopped

2 teaspoons minced garlic

1 medium stalk celery, finely chopped

2 medium carrots, peeled and chopped

1 tablespoon chili powder

1 teaspoon ground cumin

4 cups chicken bone broth

¼ teaspoon ground black pepper

3 (15-ounce) cans black beans, rinsed and drained, divided

1 (14.5-ounce) can fire-roasted diced tomatoes, drained

SERVES 8	
Per Serving:	
Calories	212
Fat	3g
Protein	15g
Sodium	521mg
Fiber	13g
Carbohydrates	32g
Net Carbs	19g
Sugar	3g

1   Heat olive oil in a large stockpot over medium heat. Add onion and garlic and cook for 3 minutes or until onion starts to soften. Add celery and carrots and cook until carrots start to soften, another 5 minutes. Stir in chili powder and cumin and cook for 1 minute.

2   Add broth, pepper, and two cans of black beans and stir. Bring to a boil over high heat and then reduce heat to low.

3   Combine remaining can of beans and fire-roasted tomatoes in a food processor and process until smooth. Pour mixture into soup and stir.

4   Cover and simmer for 30 minutes. Allow to cool slightly before serving.

Lentil and Quinoa Curry

SERVES 4

Per Serving:

Calories	450
Fat	16g
Protein	24g
Sodium	1,115mg
Fiber	13g
Carbohydrates	55g
Net Carbs	42g
Sugar	8g

This high-carbohydrate Lentil and Quinoa Curry is also packed with protein to help keep you full all day. You won't even miss the meat!

1 tablespoon olive oil

2 teaspoons minced garlic

1 small yellow onion, peeled and diced

½ cup chopped peeled carrots

1 cup sliced white mushrooms

½ cup seeded finely diced red bell pepper

4 cups chicken bone broth

1 cup dry lentils

½ cup sprouted quinoa

2 tablespoons tomato paste

1 tablespoon red chili paste

2 tablespoons curry powder

1 tablespoon ground cumin

2 teaspoons chili powder

1 teaspoon garam masala

1 teaspoon sea salt

½ teaspoon ground black pepper

¼ cup full-fat coconut milk

2 tablespoons grass-fed butter

1 Heat olive oil in a large stockpot over medium heat. Add garlic and cook for 1 minute. Add onion and cook until it starts to soften, about 4 minutes. Stir in carrots, mushrooms, and peppers and cook for 3 more minutes.

2 Stir in chicken broth, lentils, quinoa, tomato paste, red chili paste, and spices. Reduce heat to low and simmer for 1 hour. Stir in coconut milk and butter.

3 Allow to cool slightly before serving.

Apple and Beet Salad

This Apple and Beet Salad provides a boatload of nutrients, complex carbohydrates, and a deep, earthy flavor. It's a great match for any of your favorite protein dishes. Pair it with a Grilled Bison Burger (see recipe in Chapter 3) for a combination that's out of this world.

⅔ **cup apple cider vinegar**

½ **cup olive oil**

½ **teaspoon sea salt**

½ **teaspoon ground black pepper**

½ **teaspoon dry mustard**

2 **teaspoons powdered erythritol**

1 **(8.8-ounce) package cooked beets, sliced**

2 **cups arugula**

½ **small red onion, peeled and sliced into rings**

1 **Fuji apple, cored and shredded**

1 **large avocado, peeled, pitted, and diced**

½ **cup toasted pine nuts**

¼ **cup crumbled goat cheese**

1 Combine apple cider vinegar, oil, salt, pepper, mustard, and erythritol in a large bowl and whisk to incorporate. Add beets, arugula, onion, apple, avocado, and pine nuts to dressing and toss to coat.

2 Sprinkle goat cheese on top.

3 Serve immediately.

SERVES 2	
Per Serving:	
Calories	1,110
Fat	101g
Protein	14g
Sodium	980mg
Fiber	15g
Carbohydrates	47g
Net Carbs	28g
Sugar	25g

BEETS, BEETS, THE MAGICAL VEGETABLE

Beets are one of nature's miracles. According to research, when you eat beets, it can lower your blood pressure by up to 10 mm Hg in a matter of hours; it also increases your body's oxygen use by up to 20 percent, which is especially helpful before any endurance exercise. The red pigments, called *betalains*, also help reduce chronic inflammation and improve brain and gut health.

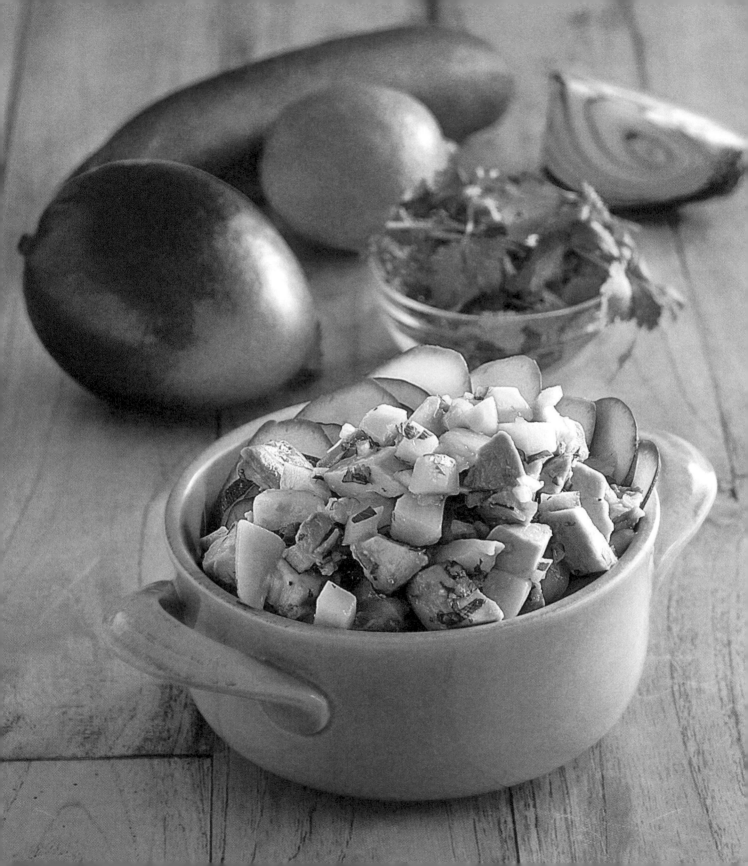

Spicy Mango Guacamole

This Spicy Mango Guacamole combines the tropical sweetness of mango with the spicy kick of a jalapeño. You can eat it with raw zucchini slices as a snack or serve it on top of Blackened Cajun Chicken (see recipe in Chapter 4).

3 large avocados, peeled, pitted, and cubed

1 medium mango, peeled and diced

1 teaspoon minced garlic

2 teaspoons chopped fresh cilantro

¼ cup finely chopped peeled red onion

2 teaspoons lime juice

¾ teaspoon sea salt

½ small jalapeño, finely diced

Place avocados in a medium mixing bowl and mash to desired consistency. Stir in remaining ingredients. Serve immediately.

SERVES 4

Per Serving:

Calories	280
Fat	23g
Protein	5g
Sodium	387mg
Fiber	6g
Carbohydrates	22g
Net Carbs	16g
Sugar	5g

KEEP YOUR EYES SHARP WITH MANGO

Mangoes are rich in many vitamins and minerals, but they're particularly loaded with zeaxanthin, an antioxidant that keeps your eyes healthy. Zeaxanthin helps filter out blue light, which is the harmful light emitted from computer screens and cell phones, and protects the eyes from developing diseases, like age-related macular degeneration.

Butternut Carrot Ginger Soup

THE APPEAL OF ORANGE VEGETABLES

Orange vegetables are most notably acclaimed for their vitamin A (more specifically, beta-carotene) content. In addition to keeping the eyes healthy, vitamin A reduces the risk of prostate cancer, lowers blood pressure, lowers cholesterol, promotes formation of collagen, boosts your immune system, and keeps your bones healthy. In addition to vitamin A, orange vegetables are also rich in lycopene, potassium, and vitamin C.

Don't let the simple ingredients fool you—this soup has a huge flavor payoff. It's also pretty forgiving, so if you don't have all the ingredients on hand, you can play around with different combinations of carrots, butternut squash, and pumpkin—three complex carbohydrates that are loaded with vitamin A.

2 tablespoons olive oil

1 teaspoon minced garlic

½ cup minced peeled yellow onion

2 tablespoons freshly grated ginger

3 cups chicken bone broth

1 cup sliced peeled carrots

1 cup cubed butternut squash

½ cup grass-fed half-and-half

¼ teaspoon ground cumin

¼ teaspoon sea salt

1 Heat oil in a medium stockpot over medium heat. Add garlic, onion, and ginger and cook for 3 minutes.

2 Add broth, carrots, and butternut squash and cover. Bring to a boil and then reduce heat to low. Simmer for 45 minutes or until carrots and squash are tender.

3 Use an immersion blender to purée mixture. Stir in half-and-half, cumin, and salt. Serve immediately.

Creamy Beet Soup

Make sure your beets are fully cooked before puréeing the soup. If you purée it too early, you'll get a grainy texture instead of a nice, smooth one.

2 tablespoons olive oil

2 teaspoons minced garlic

3 medium shallots, peeled and minced

6 medium beets, peeled and diced

2 cups chicken bone broth

1 teaspoon sea salt

½ teaspoon ground black pepper

½ teaspoon chili powder

¼ cup grass-fed half-and-half

SERVES 4	
Per Serving:	
Calories	214
Fat	9g
Protein	8g
Sodium	748mg
Fiber	5g
Carbohydrates	22g
Net Carbs	17g
Sugar	16g

1 Heat olive oil in a medium stockpot over medium heat. Add garlic and shallots and cook for 3 minutes. Add beets and cook for another 2 minutes.

2 Stir in broth, salt, pepper, and chili powder and increase heat to high. Bring to a boil, cover, and then reduce heat to low.

3 Simmer for 45 minutes or until beets are tender.

4 Use an immersion blender to purée soup to a smooth consistency. Stir in half-and-half.

5 Serve immediately.

Lentil and Sausage Soup

SERVES 4

Per Serving:

Calories	528
Fat	20g
Protein	30g
Sodium	964mg
Fiber	13g
Carbohydrates	56g
Net Carbs	43g
Sugar	20g

This hearty soup will keep you full for a long time. If you want to make a vegetarian version of it, you can omit the sausage and use vegetable broth in place of the chicken broth.

½ pound no-sugar-added hot Italian sausage

2 tablespoons olive oil

2 teaspoons minced garlic

1 large yellow onion, peeled and diced

1 medium stalk celery, diced

2 small carrots, peeled and diced

2 tablespoons tomato paste

¼ teaspoon chili powder

½ teaspoon ground cumin

½ teaspoon sea salt

¼ teaspoon ground black pepper

4 cups chicken bone broth

1 cup dry lentils

1 tablespoon lemon juice

1 Crumble sausage into a medium skillet over medium-high heat. Cook until no longer pink, about 7 minutes. Set aside.

2 Heat olive oil in a medium stockpot over medium heat. Add garlic and onions and cook for 3 minutes. Add celery and carrots and cook for 5 minutes.

3 Stir in tomato paste, chili powder, cumin, salt, and black pepper and cook for 2 more minutes.

4 Add chicken broth and lentils and stir. Increase heat to high and bring to a boil. Cover and reduce heat to low. Simmer for 30 minutes or until lentils are tender.

5 Use an immersion blender to purée soup to desired consistency. Stir in cooked sausage and lemon juice.

6 Serve immediately.

Apple Salmon Salad

This Apple Salmon Salad uses canned salmon for an added boost of omega-3 fatty acids. The shredded apples give a sweetness that complements the fish nicely and throws some complex carbohydrates in the mix.

1 (6-ounce) can wild Atlantic salmon

¼ cup keto-friendly mayonnaise

1 small Fuji apple, cored and shredded

1 tablespoon Dijon mustard

1 teaspoon fresh lemon juice

½ teaspoon sea salt

¼ teaspoon ground black pepper

SERVES 2	
Per Serving:	
Calories	379
Fat	29g
Protein	18g
Sodium	1,801mg
Fiber	2g
Carbohydrates	12g
Net Carbs	10g
Sugar	9g

1 Combine all ingredients in a medium bowl. Stir until incorporated.

2 Refrigerate for 1 hour before serving.

Sweet Potato Hummus

This variation on a basic hummus recipe adds more of a flavor boost. If the hummus comes out too thick after processing, you can thin it out by adding a little liquid from the can of garbanzo beans.

1 (15-ounce) can garbanzo beans

2 tablespoons olive oil

1 (15-ounce) can sweet potato purée

2 tablespoons tahini

2 tablespoons lemon juice

2 cloves garlic

¼ teaspoon ground cumin

¼ teaspoon ground coriander

¼ teaspoon ground black pepper

½ teaspoon sea salt

SERVES 12	
Per Serving:	
Calories	91
Fat	4g
Protein	2g
Sodium	176mg
Fiber	2g
Carbohydrates	12g
Net Carbs	10g
Sugar	3g

1 Combine garbanzo beans and oil in a food processor and pulse for 20 seconds. Add sweet potato purée and pulse for 10 seconds.

2 Add remaining ingredients and process until smooth. Refrigerate for 2 hours before serving.

Roasted Beet and Spinach Salad

SERVES 2	
Per Serving:	
Calories	258
Fat	15g
Protein	6g
Sodium	745mg
Fiber	6g
Carbohydrates	26g
Net Carbs	18g
Sugar	8g

If you want to save some time preparing this recipe, you can buy beets precooked. Try to stay away from the canned beets and instead look for the beets that are shrink-wrapped in a refrigerated part of the produce section.

1 large beet, peeled and cubed

4 teaspoons olive oil, divided

½ teaspoon sea salt

¼ teaspoon ground black pepper

1 teaspoon lemon juice

2 teaspoons Dijon mustard

¼ teaspoon minced garlic

¾ teaspoon apple cider vinegar

1 teaspoon powdered erythritol

3 cups baby spinach

2 tablespoons chopped walnuts

1 tablespoon unsweetened dried cranberries

½ cup cooked sprouted quinoa

1 Preheat oven to 350°F. Line a baking sheet with parchment paper.

2 Place cubed beets in a medium mixing bowl. Add 2 teaspoons olive oil, salt, and pepper and toss to coat. Arrange beets in a single layer on prepared baking sheet.

3 Bake for 1 hour, turning beets over once during cooking.

4 Combine remaining olive oil, lemon juice, mustard, garlic, apple cider vinegar, and erythritol in a medium bowl and whisk until smooth. Add remaining ingredients and toss to coat.

5 Add cooked beets to bowl and stir to combine. Serve immediately.

CHAPTER 12

Carb-Day Dinner

Bacon-Glazed Pork Chops with Applesauce

SLOW-COOKER APPLESAUCE

This homemade applesauce is easy to make, with only a few simple ingredients. Combine 3 pounds of sliced cored apples (keep the peel on for a true homemade feel!) with ½ cup water and 1 teaspoon ground cinnamon in a slow cooker. Cook on low for 6 hours or until soft, then use an immersion blender to purée to desired consistency. You can store it in an airtight container in the refrigerator for up to a week or in the freezer for up to 6 months.

These pork chops are deceptively simple. They don't require a lot of work or ingredients, but they taste like they just came out of the kitchen of a five-star restaurant.

½ teaspoon sea salt

¼ teaspoon ground black pepper

2 (4-ounce) boneless pork chops

1 tablespoon plus 2 teaspoons olive oil, divided

2 slices no-sugar-added bacon, chopped

¼ cup chopped peeled shallots

1 teaspoon minced garlic

1 teaspoon chicken seasoning

¼ teaspoon dried thyme

¼ cup apple cider vinegar

½ cup chicken bone broth

2 tablespoons grass-fed butter

½ cup unsweetened applesauce

1 Sprinkle salt and pepper on each pork chop and drizzle 1 teaspoon of olive oil over each chop.

2 Heat remaining olive oil in a medium cast iron skillet over medium heat. Add pork chops to hot pan and cook for 4 minutes on each side or until pork reaches desired degree of doneness.

3 Remove pork from skillet and transfer to a plate. Cover loosely with foil.

4 Add chopped bacon to pan and cook for 4 minutes. Add shallots and garlic and cook for another 2 minutes. Stir in chicken seasoning and thyme and cook for another minute.

5 Pour in vinegar and broth and stir, using a wooden spoon to scrape any browned bits off the bottom of the skillet. Reduce heat to low and cook until sauce thickens, about 4 minutes.

6 Add butter and stir until melted and smooth. Pour equal amounts of sauce over each pork chop. Scoop equal amounts of applesauce on top of each pork chop. Serve immediately.

Turkey and Quinoa Meatloaf

If you want to turn this Turkey and Quinoa Meatloaf into a convenient, portable lunch, you can shape the meat into balls and cook them in a muffin tin for 30 minutes at 350°F. Use them as a protein source to top your salads or pair them with your favorite keto-friendly side.

2 teaspoons olive oil

1 teaspoon minced garlic

1 small yellow onion, peeled and minced

½ cup chicken bone broth

¼ cup sprouted quinoa

1 pound ground turkey

1 small zucchini, minced

½ cup plus 1 tablespoon no-sugar-added ketchup, divided

2 tablespoons coconut aminos

2 large eggs

1½ teaspoons sea salt

1 teaspoon ground black pepper

2 tablespoons mustard

¼ teaspoon Worcestershire sauce

SERVES 4	
Per Serving:	
Calories	321
Fat	16g
Protein	30g
Sodium	1,300mg
Fiber	2g
Carbohydrates	17g
Net Carbs	15g
Sugar	6g

1 Heat olive oil in a medium saucepan over medium heat. Add garlic and onion and cook until softened, about 5 minutes.

2 Add chicken broth and quinoa in a medium saucepan and stir. Bring to a boil over high heat. Reduce heat to low, cover, and simmer for 15 minutes or until water is absorbed and quinoa is tender. Set aside and allow to cool.

3 Preheat oven to 350°F. Line a baking sheet with parchment paper.

4 Combine cooked quinoa, turkey, zucchini, 1 tablespoon ketchup, coconut aminos, eggs, salt, and pepper in a medium bowl and mix with your hands until thoroughly incorporated.

5 Shape mixture into a loaf on prepared baking sheet.

6 Combine remaining ketchup, mustard, and Worcestershire sauce in a small bowl and stir until smooth.

7 Spread mixture evenly on top of meatloaf.

8 Bake for 45 minutes or until no longer pink. Allow to cool before serving.

Baked Salmon with Mango Rice

CORIANDER OR CILANTRO?

Cilantro is the Spanish word for coriander, which comes from the *Coriandrum sativum* plant. In North America, *coriander* refers to the dried seeds of the plant, while *cilantro* refers to its leaves and stalks. In other parts of the world, *coriander* is the name for the leaves and stalks, while the seeds are simply called *coriander seeds*. Coriander seeds are available whole or ground and add a unique lemony citrus flavor to dishes.

You might not be on vacation, but this dish will make you feel like you are! Adding mango and coconut milk to cooked rice gives this Baked Salmon with Mango Rice a tropical feel similar to something you would find in the Caribbean.

2 teaspoons ground coriander

1 teaspoon lemon pepper

½ teaspoon sea salt

2 (4-ounce) salmon fillets

3 tablespoons grass-fed butter, divided

1 tablespoon olive oil

2 small shallots, peeled and minced

1 medium mango, peeled and finely diced

2 tablespoons unsweetened full-fat coconut milk

1 teaspoon orange zest

1 cup cooked sprouted brown rice

1 tablespoon chopped fresh cilantro

1 Preheat oven to 400°F. Line a baking sheet with parchment paper.

2 Combine coriander, lemon pepper, and salt in a small bowl and stir to incorporate.

3 Place salmon fillets skin side down on prepared baking sheet. Melt 1 tablespoon butter and brush on each fillet. Sprinkle seasoning mix on top. Bake for 20 minutes or until fish flakes easily with a fork.

4 Heat olive oil in a small saucepan over medium heat. Add shallots and cook for 2 minutes. Add mango and cook for another 2 minutes. Remove mango mixture from saucepan with a spoon and set aside.

5 Heat remaining 2 tablespoons of butter in a medium pan over medium heat. Stir in coconut milk and orange zest and bring to a boil. Stir in cooked rice and return to a boil. Reduce heat to low and stir frequently until most of the liquid is absorbed or evaporates.

6 Remove from heat and stir in mango mixture and cilantro. Divide rice mixture evenly into two portions and place each portion on a plate. Place one salmon fillet on top of each rice portion. Serve immediately.

Ground Turkey and Rice Skillet

Adding spicy kimchi sriracha makes this Ground Turkey and Rice Skillet a satisfying, low-carb dinner that's also loaded with probiotics in their most natural form.

2 tablespoons olive oil, divided

1 teaspoon minced garlic

¼ cup finely chopped peeled yellow onion

½ teaspoon paprika

1¼ cups chicken bone broth

½ cup sprouted brown rice

1 pound ground turkey

1 teaspoon granulated garlic

1 teaspoon granulated onion

½ teaspoon sea salt

¼ teaspoon ground black pepper

1 medium zucchini, diced

2 tablespoons Wildbrine Probiotic Spicy Kimchi Sriracha

SERVES 4	
Per Serving:	
Calories	383
Fat	19g
Protein	22g
Sodium	671mg
Fiber	4g
Carbohydrates	41g
Net Carbs	37g
Sugar	3g

1 Heat 1 tablespoon olive oil in a medium saucepan over medium heat. Add minced garlic and onions and cook until softened, about 5 minutes. Sprinkle paprika on top and stir.

2 Add chicken broth and rice and stir. Bring to a boil over high heat. Reduce heat to low, cover, and simmer for 45 minutes or until water is absorbed and rice is tender. Set aside and allow to cool.

3 Heat remaining olive oil in a medium skillet over medium heat. Add ground turkey and cook for 2 minutes. Stir in spices and cook for another minute. Add zucchini and cook for another 4 minutes or until turkey is no longer pink and zucchini is tender.

4 Stir in cooked rice and toss to combine.

5 Divide equally into four bowls and drizzle equal amounts of sriracha on top.

6 Serve immediately.

YOUR GUT ON KIMCHI

Kimchi is a Korean side dish made from fermented vegetables—usually cabbage. Kimchi is packed with flavor and bursting with probiotics, the good bacteria that help balance your gut. According to a report published in the *Journal of Medicinal Food*, kimchi can help fight cancer, promote a healthy weight, decrease constipation, lower cholesterol, promote brain health, boost immune function, and keep your skin healthy. That's a lot of good for only 1 gram of net carbs per 2-tablespoon serving!

Gorgonzola-Stuffed Pork Chops

If you're not a Gorgonzola person, swap it out for some feta cheese or crumbled blue cheese for equally delicious results. To boost the apple flavor of this dish, spoon a little unsweetened applesauce on top after taking the pork out of the oven.

2 tablespoons grass-fed butter

½ cup finely chopped cored Granny Smith apples

1 teaspoon dried parsley

1 teaspoon dried marjoram

1 teaspoon dried thyme

1 teaspoon ground black pepper, divided

¼ cup crumbled Gorgonzola cheese

2 (4-ounce) boneless pork chops

1 Preheat oven to 375°F.

2 Heat butter in a small skillet over medium heat. Add apples, parsley, marjoram, thyme, and ¼ teaspoon black pepper and stir to combine. Cook, stirring occasionally, for 15 minutes or until apples are softened.

3 Transfer apple mixture to a small bowl and stir in Gorgonzola cheese. Set aside.

4 Cut a slit into each pork chop and put half of the apple mixture into each slit. Secure with a toothpick. Sprinkle remaining black pepper on pork chops.

5 Bake for 1 hour or until pork is no longer pink in the center.

6 Remove from oven and allow to cool before serving.

Roasted Chicken with Beets and Sweets

This recipe combines lean protein with two different types of complex carbohydrates to give you the carbs you need while also maximizing your micronutrient intake. Serve it with a side salad to get those greens in!

1 (4.5-pound) whole chicken

2 tablespoons olive oil, divided

2 teaspoons minced garlic

1 teaspoon paprika

6 medium beets, peeled and cubed

3 small sweet potatoes, peeled and cubed

1 teaspoon granulated garlic

1 teaspoon sea salt

½ teaspoon ground black pepper

1 large sweet onion, peeled and roughly chopped

1 Preheat oven to 400°F.

2 Arrange chicken in a large roasting pan. Brush 1 tablespoon olive oil all over chicken and rub with garlic. Sprinkle paprika on top.

3 Combine beets and potatoes in a large mixing bowl. Add remaining olive oil, granulated garlic, salt, and pepper and toss to coat evenly. Arrange seasoned beets and potatoes around chicken in pan.

4 Arrange chopped onion on beets and sweet potatoes.

5 Bake for 1 hour or until chicken reaches 165°F. Remove from oven and allow to rest for 10 minutes before slicing chicken.

6 Slice and serve.

SERVES 6	
Per Serving:	
Calories	486
Fat	26g
Protein	44g
Sodium	543mg
Fiber	4g
Carbohydrates	18g
Net Carbs	14g
Sugar	9g

Spinach and Goat Cheese Flank Steak Pinwheels

MAKING YOUR OWN GARLIC PASTE

Most grocery stores have garlic paste available in the refrigerator of the produce section, near the packaged herbs. If you can't find any, you can make your own with two basic ingredients: garlic and salt. Mince your garlic, sprinkle sea salt on top, and then use a chef's knife to mash, flatten, and scrape it together until a paste forms. Three cloves of garlic and ½ teaspoon of salt make about a tablespoon of garlic paste.

If you're not a fan of goat cheese, you can replace it with an equal amount of feta cheese or blue cheese. You can also add cooked, crumbled bacon to the spinach mixture to up the fat content and the smoky, salty flavor.

¼ cup olive oil

¼ cup coconut aminos

¼ cup keto-friendly red wine

¼ cup Worcestershire sauce

1 tablespoon Dijon mustard

2 cloves minced garlic

1 teaspoon Italian seasoning

½ teaspoon ground black pepper

1½ pounds flank steak

1 cup frozen chopped spinach, thawed and drained

½ cup crumbled goat cheese

½ teaspoon sea salt

2 tablespoons garlic paste

1 Combine olive oil, coconut aminos, wine, Worcestershire sauce, mustard, minced garlic, Italian seasoning, and black pepper in a large resealable plastic bag. Pierce flank steak with knife, place in bag, and seal.

2 Massage steak to work marinade into it and refrigerate 8 hours or overnight.

3 Preheat oven to 350°F.

4 Combine spinach, goat cheese, and salt in a small bowl. Set aside.

5 Pound steak out to ½-inch thickness. Spread garlic paste on steak. Spoon spinach mixture on top of garlic.

6 Roll steak up lengthwise and secure with toothpicks. Place in a 9" × 13" baking dish.

7 Cook for 1 hour or until internal temperature reaches 145°F. Remove from oven and let meat sit for 10 minutes before slicing. Serve warm.

Creamy Chicken and Wild Rice Soup

If you want to enjoy this soup on one of your low-carb days, you can replace the rice with cauliflower rice and use a few teaspoons of arrowroot powder in place of the flour. You can also swap out the coconut milk for heavy cream if you want a thicker soup with extra fat.

3 cups chicken bone broth

1½ cups water

3 cups shredded cooked chicken

3 cups cooked wild rice

½ cup paleo flour

¼ teaspoon sea salt

¼ teaspoon ground black pepper

¼ cup grass-fed butter

1 tablespoon chicken seasoning

1½ cups full-fat coconut milk

SERVES 6	
Per Serving:	
Calories	438
Fat	25g
Protein	30g
Sodium	924mg
Fiber	3g
Carbohydrates	24g
Net Carbs	21g
Sugar	2g

1 Combine broth and water in a large stockpot over medium-high heat. Bring to a boil, stir in chicken and rice, and reduce heat to low.

2 Combine flour, salt, and pepper in a small bowl. Heat butter in a small saucepan over medium heat. Add chicken seasoning and stir to incorporate. Reduce heat to low. Slowly stir in seasoned flour.

3 Pour coconut milk into flour mixture slowly, whisking until smooth. Cook for 5 minutes or until mixture thickens.

4 Add mixture to stockpot and stir to combine. Cook for 10 minutes. Remove from heat and serve.

Mexican Quinoa Skillet

SERVES 4

Per Serving:

Calories	401
Fat	11g
Protein	26g
Sodium	799mg
Fiber	12g
Carbohydrates	55g
Net Carbs	43g
Sugar	6g

This Mexican Quinoa Skillet is an easy one-pan dish that's quick to whip up on a busy weeknight. You can add some variation to it by incorporating some different vegetables, like red bell pepper or sweet potato, and switching up the meat—lime chicken and shrimp work well too!

1 teaspoon crushed red pepper

2 teaspoons chili powder

¾ teaspoon cumin

¼ teaspoon paprika

¼ teaspoon granulated garlic

¼ teaspoon granulated onion

¼ teaspoon dried oregano

½ teaspoon sea salt

¼ teaspoon ground black pepper

1 tablespoon avocado oil

1 small jalapeño, seeded and minced

1 teaspoon minced garlic

½ pound ground turkey

1 (14.5-ounce) can fire-roasted tomatoes, drained

1 (15-ounce) can black beans, rinsed and drained

1 cup sprouted quinoa, rinsed

1 cup chicken bone broth

¼ cup chopped fresh cilantro

1 Combine spices in a small bowl. Set aside.

2 Heat avocado oil in a medium skillet over medium heat. Add jalapeño and minced garlic and cook for 2 minutes. Stir in ground turkey and spices and cook until no longer pink, about 7 minutes.

3 Add remaining ingredients, except cilantro, and stir to combine. Bring to a boil, then reduce heat to low. Cover and cook for 15 minutes or until quinoa is tender and most of the liquid is absorbed.

4 Remove from heat and stir in cilantro. Serve warm.

Curried Chicken and Brown Rice

If you don't have sprouted rice, you can use any brown rice you have. If grains bother your stomach at all, it's worth the extra effort to buy sprouted rice or to sprout it yourself.

2 tablespoons coconut oil, divided

½ cup chopped peeled yellow onion

1 teaspoon minced garlic

1 cup sprouted brown rice

1½ teaspoons sea salt, divided

1 teaspoon curry powder

1 teaspoon garam masala

½ teaspoon ground cumin

2 cups chicken bone broth

12 ounces boneless, skinless chicken breasts, cubed

½ teaspoon chicken seasoning

¼ teaspoon ground black pepper

1 Heat 1 tablespoon coconut oil in a medium saucepan over medium heat. Add onion and garlic and cook for 2 minutes. Stir in rice, ½ teaspoon salt, curry powder, garam masala, and cumin. Cook for another minute.

2 Pour chicken broth into pan, stir, and bring to a boil. Reduce heat to low, add rice, cover, and cook for 45 minutes or until rice is tender and liquid is absorbed.

3 While rice is cooking, heat remaining coconut oil in a medium skillet over medium heat. Add chicken and cook for 2 minutes. Add remaining salt, chicken seasoning, and pepper and cook until chicken is no longer pink, about 5 more minutes.

4 Add cooked rice to skillet and toss to combine. Serve warm.

SERVES 4

Per Serving:

Calories	348
Fat	11g
Protein	26g
Sodium	1,210mg
Fiber	3g
Carbohydrates	37g
Net Carbs	34g
Sugar	1g

SPROUTED RICE

Antinutrients are natural compounds within grains that protect the plant from animals and insects. The purpose of antinutrients is to make anyone or anything who eats the plants feel a little sick—with the goal that they'll learn and stop eating the plant. Antinutrients also bind to vitamins, minerals, and amino acids so that you can't absorb them properly and inhibit your own digestive enzymes, which makes it harder to break down the grains. Sprouting, which involves soaking grains in water until they germinate, can reduce antinutrients.

Roasted Beets

Per Serving:

Calories	67
Fat	4g
Protein	1g
Sodium	400mg
Fiber	2g
Carbohydrates	6g
Net Carbs	4g
Sugar	4g

SAUTÉED BEET GREENS

Beet greens are a rich source of zeaxanthin—a carotenoid that keeps your eyes healthy and helps protect against age-related macular degeneration. To make sautéed beet greens, add greens and ½ teaspoon sea salt to a medium pot of boiling water. Blanch for 2 minutes, then transfer to a bowl of ice water. Heat 2 tablespoons avocado oil in a medium skillet over medium-high heat. Add 2 minced garlic cloves, blanched beet greens, ½ teaspoon sea salt, ¼ teaspoon crushed red pepper, and ¼ teaspoon black pepper and cook for 3 minutes.

When working with fresh beets, many people use the beet and discard the greens, but if you're doing this, you're missing out on valuable nutrients. Save the beet greens and use them to make another low-carb side dish for your next meal (see sidebar).

1 tablespoon olive oil

1 tablespoon grass-fed butter, melted

2 teaspoons minced garlic

1 bunch of beets, greens removed and peeled

1 teaspoon sea salt

½ teaspoon ground black pepper

1 Preheat oven to 350°F. Line a baking sheet with parchment paper.

2 Combine olive oil, butter, and minced garlic in a small bowl and pour over beets. Toss to coat.

3 Spread beets on prepared baking sheet, sprinkle with salt and pepper, and roast for 1 hour or until a knife slides through beets easily.

4 Cool slightly, then slice beets and serve.

Cinnamon Apple Pork Chops

These Cinnamon Apple Pork Chops are full of flavor and very tender. If you want to increase the sweetness a little bit, use Fuji or Gala apples in place of the Granny Smith apples.

½ teaspoon sea salt

¼ teaspoon ground black pepper

4 (4-ounce) boneless pork chops

¼ cup grass-fed butter

2 tablespoons golden monk fruit sweetener

½ teaspoon ground cinnamon

½ teaspoon ground nutmeg

2 teaspoons arrowroot powder

1 tablespoon water

4 Granny Smith apples, peeled, cored, and diced

SERVES 4	
Per Serving:	
Calories	381
Fat	16g
Protein	27g
Sodium	336mg
Fiber	5g
Carbohydrates	42g
Net Carbs	31g
Sugar	25g

1 Preheat oven to 350°F.

2 Sprinkle salt and pepper all over pork chops and transfer chops to a 9" × 13" baking dish.

3 Heat butter in a medium saucepan over medium heat. Stir in sweetener, cinnamon, and nutmeg and reduce heat to low.

4 Mix arrowroot powder with water in a small bowl, then add to sauce. Stir in apples.

5 Simmer for 10 minutes or until sauce thickens.

6 Pour sauce over pork chops and bake for 35 minutes or until pork chops reach desired level of doneness. Serve warm.

Blackened Salmon and Mango Salsa

SERVES 4	
Per Serving:	
Calories	411
Fat	19g
Protein	22g
Sodium	1,153mg
Fiber	6g
Carbohydrates	43g
Net Carbs	37g
Sugar	35g

If you want to make this dish for one of your low-carb days, replace the mangoes with avocados for a creamy, fat-rich salsa. Add a drizzle of Tessemae's Organic Habanero Ranch Dressing to finish it off.

Mango Salsa

3 medium mangoes, peeled and diced

1 small jalapeño, finely minced

2 tablespoons lime juice

2 tablespoons chopped fresh cilantro

⅛ teaspoon sea salt

Blackened Salmon

2 tablespoons ground paprika

1 tablespoon cayenne pepper

1 tablespoon onion powder

2 teaspoons sea salt

1 teaspoon ground black pepper

¼ teaspoon dried thyme

¼ teaspoon dried basil

¼ teaspoon dried oregano

2 tablespoons olive oil

4 (4-ounce) salmon fillets, skin removed

1 **For Mango Salsa:** Combine mangoes, jalapeño, lime juice, cilantro, and salt in a medium bowl and mix to incorporate. Place in the refrigerator while salmon cooks.

2 **For Blackened Salmon:** Preheat oven to broil. Line a baking sheet with parchment paper.

3 Combine paprika, cayenne pepper, onion powder, salt, black pepper, thyme, basil, and oregano in a small bowl.

4 Rub olive oil on both sides of salmon and coat salmon in seasoning mixture.

5 Arrange salmon on prepared baking sheet. Broil for 3 minutes per side or until fish flakes apart easily with a fork.

6 When salmon is done cooking, top each fillet with equal amounts of Mango Salsa. Serve immediately.

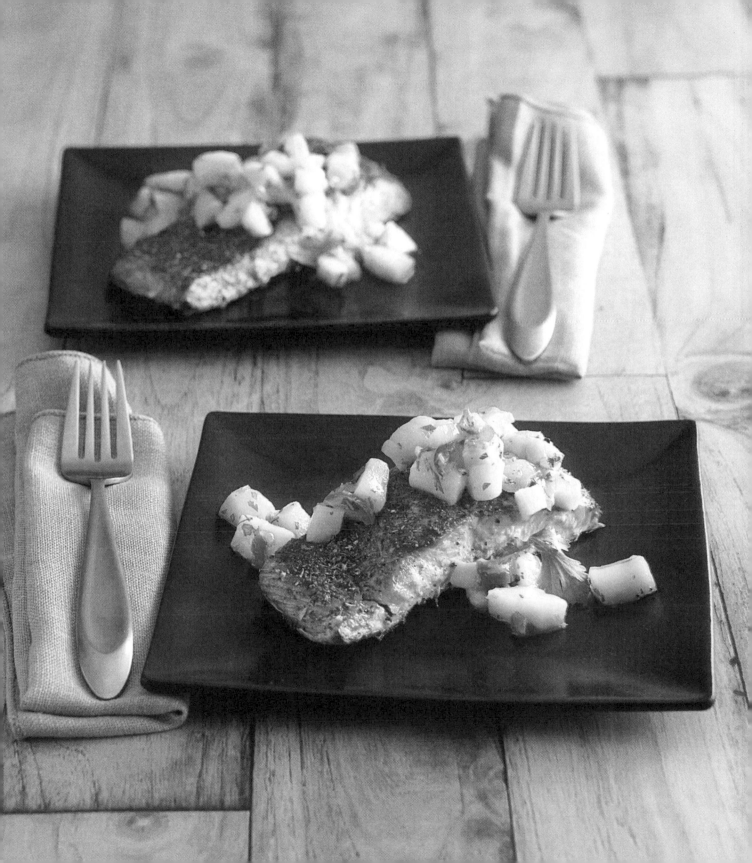

Spicy Basil Chicken and Rice

THAI BASIL VERSUS ITALIAN BASIL

Thai basil is a variety of the sweet Italian basil you typically see but with a vastly different flavor profile. Thai basil has a spicy, licorice-like (or anise) flavor, while Italian basil has a sweet, peppery taste. It also stands up to heat, unlike Italian basil, so you can use it during cooking, rather than adding it in at the end. Thai basil has a unique taste and brings an authentic flavor profile to Thai dishes, so if you can find it, use it!

You may not be able to find some of the ingredients (bird's eye chilis and Thai basil) at your regular supermarket. If you can't, try your local Asian market!

1 teaspoon powdered monk fruit sweetener

⅓ cup fish sauce

¼ cup avocado oil

2 teaspoons minced garlic

3 bird's eye (Thai) chilis, minced

1 large red bell pepper, seeded and thinly sliced

1 medium yellow onion, peeled and thinly sliced

2 tablespoons coconut aminos

1 pound ground chicken

3 cups cooked sprouted brown rice

2 scallions, diced

2 cups chopped Thai basil

1 Combine sweetener and fish sauce in a small bowl and whisk together.

2 Heat avocado oil in a medium skillet over medium-high heat. Add garlic, bird's eye chilis, bell pepper, and onion and stir to avoid burning. Stir in fish sauce mixture and coconut aminos and cook for 2 minutes.

3 Add chicken and cook until no longer pink, about 7 minutes.

4 Stir in rice and scallions. Remove from heat and stir in basil.

5 Serve warm.

Chicken Fried Rice

Although peas don't fit into a strict keto diet, they're actually a healthy carbohydrate choice for your higher-carb days. Keep frozen peas in your freezer and add them to recipes whenever you need a carbohydrate boost.

2 tablespoons avocado oil, divided

½ cup chopped peeled sweet onion

2 teaspoons minced garlic

1 small red bell pepper, seeded and chopped

12 ounces boneless, skinless chicken breasts, cut into strips

2 cups cooked sprouted brown rice

2 tablespoons coconut aminos

1 tablespoon rice vinegar

1 cup frozen peas, thawed

1 Heat 1 tablespoon avocado oil in a medium skillet over medium heat. Add onion and garlic and cook for 2 minutes. Add bell pepper and cook for another minute.

2 Stir in chicken and cook until chicken is no longer pink, about 7 minutes. Remove chicken from pan and set aside.

3 Heat remaining avocado oil in skillet and add remaining ingredients. Stir to combine. Add chicken to mixture and cook for 1 more minute or until heated through.

4 Remove from heat and serve warm.

SERVES 4

Per Serving:

Calories	324
Fat	11g
Protein	22g
Sodium	425mg
Fiber	4g
Carbohydrates	33g
Net Carbs	29g
Sugar	5g

DESCRIPTION OF PEAS

One cup of peas contains 21 grams of carbohydrates. While around 8 grams of those carbohydrates come from fiber, the rest come from starches and natural sugars. Although classified as legumes, peas are botanically more like a fruit. Unlike other legumes, peas are low in phytates and lectins, the two antinutrients that make digesting legumes difficult. Because of this, peas are often touted as one of the better legume choices.

Quinoa and Black Bean–Stuffed Peppers

SERVES 4	
Per Serving:	
Calories	433
Fat	9g
Protein	22g
Sodium	1,039mg
Fiber	14g
Carbohydrates	69g
Net Carbs	55g
Sugar	11g

These Quinoa and Black Bean–Stuffed Peppers don't need any meat—they're full of protein and completely satisfying without it; but if you want to add some, cook it before adding it to the stuffing mixture.

1½ cups chicken bone broth

1 cup sprouted quinoa, rinsed

4 large red bell peppers

1½ cups no-sugar-added salsa, divided

1 (15-ounce) can black beans, rinsed and drained

½ cup full-fat cottage cheese, divided

½ cup shredded Cheddar cheese, divided

2 teaspoons keto-friendly taco seasoning

1 Preheat oven to 375°F.

2 Add chicken broth and quinoa in a medium saucepan and stir. Bring to a boil over high heat. Reduce heat to low, cover, and simmer for 15 minutes or until water is absorbed and quinoa is tender. Set aside and allow to cool.

3 Cut tops off peppers and remove seeds. Arrange in a baking dish, cut side up.

4 Combine cooked quinoa, 1 cup salsa, black beans, cottage cheese, ¼ cup Cheddar cheese, and taco seasoning in a medium bowl and stir until smooth.

5 Spoon equal amounts of mixture into each bell pepper. Spoon remaining salsa and sprinkle remaining cheese on top.

6 Bake for 35 minutes or until peppers are slightly softened and stuffing is heated through. Serve warm.

Spicy Sausage and White Bean Soup

White beans add lots of fiber to this soup. Since fiber is something that can be hard to get during your low-carb days, load up on your higher-carb days to keep your digestive system running smoothly.

1 tablespoon olive oil

1 pound no-sugar-added pork sausage

1 large yellow onion, peeled and diced

2 tablespoons minced garlic

4 cups chicken bone broth

½ cup keto-friendly white wine

2 cups frozen chopped spinach

¼ cup chopped fresh parsley

2 (15-ounce) cans cannellini beans, rinsed and drained

1 teaspoon sea salt

1 teaspoon ground black pepper

½ teaspoon crushed red pepper

1 Heat olive oil in a medium skillet over medium heat. Add sausage and cook until browned, about 5 minutes. Add onion and garlic and cook until softened, about 3 minutes. Transfer to a slow cooker.

2 Add remaining ingredients and stir. Cover and cook on low for 4 hours.

3 Remove from heat and serve warm.

SERVES 4

Per Serving:

Calories	1177
Fat	64g
Protein	80g
Sodium	1,529mg
Fiber	20g
Carbohydrates	67g
Net Carbs	47g
Sugar	7g

EASY PORK SAUSAGE

It's difficult to find premade sausage that doesn't have added sugar. Even though the carbohydrates might fit into your high-carb days, sugar isn't a good place to get them. Fortunately, it's easy to make your own sausage without it. In a small bowl, combine 1 teaspoon salt, ½ teaspoon dried parsley, ¼ teaspoon ground sage, ¼ teaspoon black pepper, ¼ teaspoon dried thyme, ¼ teaspoon crushed red pepper, ⅛ teaspoon cayenne pepper, and ¼ teaspoon ground coriander. Mix thoroughly into 1 pound ground pork before cooking.

Chicken Sausage with Sweet Potato Noodles

Per Serving:

Calories	315
Fat	20g
Protein	16g
Sodium	1,350mg
Fiber	4g
Carbohydrates	20g
Net Carbs	16g
Sugar	5g

This recipe is sinfully easy. All it takes is a few ingredients and a few minutes of cooking time, and you'll have a meal on your table in minutes. If you don't have a vegetable spiralizer, you can chop the sweet potatoes instead, but you'll have to adjust the cooking time.

2 tablespoons grass-fed butter

½ cup frozen chopped spinach, thawed

2 no-sugar-added chicken and apple sausage links, cut into half-moons

1 large sweet potato, spiralized

½ teaspoon sea salt

⅛ teaspoon ground cinnamon

1 Heat butter in a medium skillet over medium heat. Add spinach and cook until heated through, about 3 minutes. Add sausage links and cook until heated through and browned, about 5 minutes.

2 Add sweet potato noodles, salt, and cinnamon and stir to combine. Cover and cook for 3 minutes. Stir, cover, and cook for another 3 minutes or until noodles are tender.

3 Remove from heat and serve.

Salmon Florentine

White wine is naturally low in carbohydrates—a 5-ounce serving contains only 3.8 grams. Although technically low in carbs, it's not the best beverage choice on a keto diet, but you can use it occasionally for cooking.

½ cup grass-fed butter

1 small white onion, peeled and sliced

2 teaspoons minced garlic

4 (4-ounce) salmon fillets, skin removed

¾ cup keto-friendly dry white wine

¾ cup grass-fed half-and-half

¼ teaspoon sea salt

¼ teaspoon ground black pepper

3 cups chopped spinach

2 cups cooked brown rice

1 Heat butter in a medium skillet over medium-high heat. Add onion and garlic and cook for 5 minutes.

2 Add salmon to skillet and cook for 2 minutes. Pour wine and half-and-half over salmon and stir carefully. Add salt and pepper and cover.

3 Cook for 7 minutes, remove cover, stir spinach into cream mixture carefully, and flip salmon over. Cook for another 7 minutes or until salmon flakes apart easily with a fork.

4 Remove from heat and serve over rice.

SERVES 4	
Per Serving:	
Calories	596
Fat	40g
Protein	24g
Sodium	234mg
Fiber	3g
Carbohydrates	32g
Net Carbs	29g
Sugar	3g

IS WINE KETO-FRIENDLY?

Drinking alcohol messes with your blood sugar and can kick you out of ketosis, no matter how many carbohydrates your drink contains. It's best to stay away from it as a beverage choice if you want some serious results on your keto cycling plan. That being said, you can cook with wine occasionally. Most of the alcohol burns off during cooking, although the carbs are still there. Choose your cooking wines wisely—white wines are lower in carbs than red wines.

Stuffed Sweet Potatoes

SERVES 2	
Per Serving:	
Calories	390
Fat	20g
Protein	26g
Sodium	1,200mg
Fiber	4g
Carbohydrates	26g
Net Carbs	22g
Sugar	5g

These Stuffed Sweet Potatoes are simple and delicious. You can have them ready to eat in just about 30 minutes, making them a perfect weeknight meal. If you have room for extra fat in your daily macronutrient breakdown, you can top them with some sliced avocado or a drizzle of ranch dressing.

1 large sweet potato, cut in half lengthwise

1 tablespoon olive oil

½ pound 85/15 ground beef

1 teaspoon onion powder

1 teaspoon garlic powder

1 teaspoon sea salt

1 teaspoon ground black pepper

½ teaspoon chili powder

1 cup chopped spinach

¼ teaspoon ground cinnamon

1 Preheat oven to 375°F. Line a baking sheet with parchment paper.

2 Place sweet potato, cut side down, on prepared baking sheet and bake for 25 minutes or until sweet potato is soft. Remove from heat.

3 Heat olive oil in a medium skillet over medium heat. Add beef, onion powder, garlic powder, salt, pepper, and chili powder and cook until beef is no longer pink, about 7 minutes. Stir in spinach.

4 Place one half of each sweet potato on a plate. Mash with a fork and sprinkle cinnamon on top. Mash again to combine.

5 Scoop equal amounts of mixture into each half. Serve warm.

Spicy Lentil Chili

You can make this Spicy Lentil Chili with any protein addition that sounds good to you. Ground turkey, ground chicken, ground beef, turkey sausage, and pork sausage all work. Rotate through them every time you make it for some easy variety in your keto cycling plan.

1 cup dry lentils

4 cups chicken bone broth

1 tablespoon olive oil

1 teaspoon minced garlic

1 small yellow onion, peeled and chopped

1 medium jalapeño, minced

2 medium stalks celery, chopped

1 large red bell pepper, seeded and diced

1 pound ground turkey

1 (15-ounce) can petite-diced tomatoes, drained

1 (4-ounce) can diced green chilis

1 teaspoon ground turmeric

1 teaspoon ground cumin

1 teaspoon sea salt

1 teaspoon chili powder

½ teaspoon ground black pepper

¼ teaspoon crushed red pepper

SERVES 4	
Per Serving:	
Calories	440
Fat	13g
Protein	45g
Sodium	1,285mg
Fiber	12g
Carbohydrates	42g
Net Carbs	30g
Sugar	7g

1 Combine lentils and broth in a large stockpot over high heat. Bring to a boil, reduce heat to medium-low, and simmer for 10 minutes.

2 Heat olive oil in a medium skillet over medium heat. Add garlic, onion, and jalapeño and cook for 2 minutes. Add celery and bell pepper and cook for another 2 minutes. Crumble turkey into pan and cook until no longer pink, about 7 minutes.

3 Stir in remaining ingredients and cook for 5 more minutes.

4 Transfer turkey mixture to pot with lentils and stir to combine. Allow to simmer for another 30 minutes or until lentils are tender.

5 Remove from heat and serve.

Beet and Beef Soup

Beets and beef may not be a combo that you're used to, but they're an underrated pair. The beef soaks up the sweet earthiness of the beets, making this hearty soup something that will become part of your regular rotation.

SERVES 4	
Per Serving:	
Calories	509
Fat	23g
Protein	52g
Sodium	2,295mg
Fiber	4g
Carbohydrates	18g
Net Carbs	14g
Sugar	12g

HOMEMADE STEAK SEASONING

Most commercial steak seasonings have added oils, flavorings, sugar, and other artificial ingredients that you probably don't want in your food. Make your own version by combining 1 tablespoon paprika, 1 tablespoon ground black pepper, 1 tablespoon sea salt, 1½ teaspoons granulated garlic, 1½ teaspoons granulation onion, 1½ teaspoons ground coriander, 1½ teaspoons dried dill, and 1½ teaspoons crushed red pepper. Store in an airtight container for up to 6 months.

2 tablespoons olive oil

1 pound beef stew meat

1 small yellow onion, peeled and chopped

3 medium carrots, peeled and finely chopped

¼ cup chopped celery

6 cups beef bone broth

3 bay leaves

4 beets, peeled and cubed

1 cup chopped red cabbage

3 teaspoons keto-friendly steak seasoning

2 tablespoons white vinegar

1½ teaspoons sea salt

1 teaspoon ground black pepper

½ cup full-fat plain yogurt

1 Heat olive oil in a large stockpot over medium-high heat. Add stew meat and cook for 5 minutes, browning on all sides. Add onions, carrots, and celery and cook for 3 more minutes.

2 Stir in beef broth, bay leaves, beets, cabbage, and steak seasoning. Simmer for 1 hour or until beef is cooked through and vegetables are tender.

3 Stir in vinegar, salt, and pepper. Remove from heat, remove bay leaves, and serve with yogurt on top.

Cashew Rice Pilaf

This Cashew Rice Pilaf is the perfect high-carb side dish for any of your favorite lean protein meals. Combine it with chicken, beef, or fish or add some shrimp right to it if you want to make a one-pan dinner.

2 tablespoons grass-fed butter

2 tablespoons minced peeled yellow onion

½ teaspoon minced garlic

½ cup sprouted brown rice

2 tablespoons broken pieces brown rice spaghetti

1¼ cups chicken bone broth

½ teaspoon sea salt

½ teaspoon ground black pepper

¼ cup halved cashews

1 Heat butter in a medium saucepan over medium-low heat. Add onion and garlic and cook for 2 minutes. Add brown rice and cook for 5 minutes. Stir in spaghetti pieces and cook for 1 more minute.

2 Stir in broth, salt, and pepper and increase heat to medium-high. Bring to a boil, cover, reduce heat to low, and cook for 45 minutes or until rice is cooked and liquid is absorbed.

3 Remove from heat and fluff with a fork. Stir in cashews and serve.

SERVES 2

Per Serving:

Calories	480
Fat	27g
Protein	12g
Sodium	706mg
Fiber	4g
Carbohydrates	50g
Net Carbs	46g
Sugar	2g

BENEFITS OF CASHEWS

Cashews are one of the highest-carbohydrate nuts, containing 8.5 grams per ounce, only about 1 gram of which comes from fiber. In addition to providing complex carbohydrates, cashews also contain vitamin E, vitamin K, vitamin B_6, copper, zinc, magnesium, iron, and selenium. Cashews also contain high levels of lutein and zeaxanthin, two antioxidants that keep your eyes healthy.

Sweet Potato Chili

SERVES 6

Per Serving:

Calories	610
Fat	25g
Protein	34g
Sodium	1,396mg
Fiber	19g
Carbohydrates	64g
Net Carbs	45g
Sugar	21g

The cinnamon in this Sweet Potato Chili adds a subtle sweet under-tone that complements the natural sweetness of the sweet pota-toes, while the fire-roasted tomatoes and chili powder add that little kick that makes a chili a chili.

1 tablespoon olive oil

2 teaspoons minced garlic

1 large sweet onion, peeled and chopped

½ cup chopped seeded orange bell pepper

½ pound 85/15 ground beef

½ pound ground pork

2 medium sweet potatoes, peeled and diced

1 (14.5-ounce) can fire-roasted tomatoes, drained

1 (14.5-ounce) can petite-diced tomatoes, drained

1 (8-ounce) can tomato sauce

1 (4-ounce) can tomato paste

½ cup beef bone broth

1 (15-ounce) can black beans, rinsed and drained

1½ tablespoons chili powder

1½ teaspoons ground cumin

⅛ teaspoon cayenne pepper

½ teaspoon sea salt

½ teaspoon ground black pepper

½ teaspoon ground cinnamon

1 Heat olive oil in a large stockpot over medium heat. Add garlic and onion and cook for 2 minutes. Add bell pepper and cook for another 3 minutes. Crumble beef and pork into mixture and cook until no longer pink, about 7 minutes.

2 Stir in remaining ingredients, partially cover, and reduce heat to low. Simmer for 90 minutes or until sweet potatoes are tender and flavors have melded together, stirring occasionally.

3 Serve warm.

Moroccan Ground Beef with Lentils

If you don't have a pressure cooker, you can make this Moroccan Ground Beef with Lentils on the stovetop by letting it simmer for 20 minutes or until the lentils are tender.

1 tablespoon olive oil

1 pound 85/15 ground beef

2 teaspoons minced garlic

1 large yellow onion, peeled and diced

1 medium stalk celery, diced

3 medium carrots, peeled and shredded

1 teaspoon ground cumin

1 teaspoon ground cinnamon

½ teaspoon ground coriander

½ teaspoon turmeric

¼ teaspoon ground ginger

¼ teaspoon crushed red pepper

½ teaspoon sea salt

½ teaspoon ground black pepper

2 cups beef bone broth

1 (14.5-ounce) can petite-diced tomatoes, drained

1 (14.5-ounce) fire-roasted diced tomatoes, drained

2 tablespoons tomato paste

1 cup dry lentils

SERVES 4

Per Serving:

Calories	563
Fat	20g
Protein	45g
Sodium	1,048mg
Fiber	14g
Carbohydrates	49g
Net Carbs	35g
Sugar	11g

1 Set your pressure cooker to the sauté function. Add oil to pot and crumble ground beef into it. Add garlic, onion, celery, and carrots and cook until beef is no longer pink, about 7 minutes.

2 Add remaining ingredients to pot and stir to combine.

3 Cover pot and seal. Choose the soup setting on your pressure cooker and set for 10 minutes. Allow pressure to release naturally.

4 Remove lid and allow to cool slightly before serving.

HEALTH BENEFITS OF LENTILS

Lentils come in several different varieties—brown, red, green, yellow, and black. No matter which color you pick, lentils are an excellent source of protein. About 26 percent of the calories in lentils comes from protein. They're also loaded with complex carbohydrates that provide a sustained source of energy. Studies show that eating lentils can help lower cholesterol, reduce your risk of heart disease, prevent constipation, and stabilize blood sugar.

Ground Turkey and Garbanzo Beans

SERVES 4

Per Serving:

Calories	379
Fat	15g
Protein	34g
Sodium	1,074mg
Fiber	10g
Carbohydrates	36g
Net Carbs	26g
Sugar	10g

ANOTHER FIBER-RICH LEGUME

Garbanzo beans, also called *chickpeas*, are classified as legumes, along with beans and peanuts. Although garbanzo beans are high in carbohydrates, they're also full of fiber, which means they move through your digestive system slowly and don't have dramatic effects on your blood sugar levels. Because of this, they're a great way to get carbohydrates on your high-carb days. One cup of garbanzo beans contains 44 grams of carbohydrates, 12 grams of which come from fiber.

This recipe is a meal on its own, but if you want to up the carbohydrate count and make it a little heartier, you can serve it over cooked rice.

1 tablespoon olive oil

1 teaspoon minced garlic

1 medium yellow onion, peeled and chopped

1 pound ground turkey

1 (15-ounce) can garbanzo beans

1 (15-ounce) can tomato sauce

1 tablespoon tomato paste

1 teaspoon dried oregano

½ teaspoon sea salt

¼ teaspoon ground black pepper

1 teaspoon ground cumin

½ teaspoon cayenne pepper

¼ cup chopped fresh parsley

1 Heat olive oil in a large skillet over medium heat. Add garlic and onion and cook until softened, about 3 minutes.

2 Add turkey and cook until no longer pink, about 7 minutes. Stir in remaining ingredients, except parsley, and bring to a boil.

3 Reduce heat to low and simmer for 45 minutes or until sauce thickens. Remove from heat, stir in parsley, and serve.

Sweet Potato Enchilada Skillet

This Sweet Potato Enchilada Skillet is the perfect combination of natural sweetness and spicy. You can finish it off with some chopped fresh cilantro, some black olives, a dollop of sour cream, or some sliced avocado.

SERVES 4

Per Serving:

Calories	458
Fat	25g
Protein	30g
Sodium	692mg
Fiber	6g
Carbohydrates	30g
Net Carbs	24g
Sugar	13g

Enchilada Sauce

1 tablespoon coconut oil

¼ cup chopped peeled yellow onion

1 (14-ounce) can tomato sauce

2 tablespoons tomato paste

⅓ cup chicken bone broth

½ teaspoon granulated garlic

½ teaspoon dried oregano

½ teaspoon chili powder

½ teaspoon sea salt

½ teaspoon ground black pepper

Sweet Potato Mixture

2 tablespoons coconut oil

2 medium sweet potatoes, peeled and shredded

1 pound 85/15 ground beef

⅓ cup chopped peeled yellow onion

1 teaspoon minced garlic

1 (4-ounce) can diced green chilis

½ teaspoon chili powder

½ teaspoon ground cumin

¼ teaspoon sea salt

¼ teaspoon ground black pepper

1 **For Enchilada Sauce:** Heat coconut oil in a medium saucepan over medium heat. Add onion and cook until softened, about 3 minutes. Add remaining ingredients and stir until smooth. Reduce heat to low and simmer for 10 minutes or until thickened.

2 **For Sweet Potato Mixture:** Heat coconut oil in a medium skillet over medium heat. Add sweet potatoes and cook for 3 minutes. Crumble ground beef into the mixture and cook for 2 minutes. Add remaining ingredients, stir to incorporate, and cook until beef is no longer pink, about 5 more minutes.

3 Pour sauce over sweet potato mixture and stir to combine. Remove from heat and serve.

Keto Cycling Menus

Two High-Carb Days

	M	T	W	T	F	S	S
	Standard Keto Diet	Standard Keto Diet	Standard Keto Diet	Standard Keto Diet	Standard Keto Diet	**High-Carb Phase**	**High-Carb Phase**
Breakfast	Avocado Everything "Bagels"	Chocolate Coffee Chia Pudding	Buffalo Chicken Egg Cups	Chocolate Chip Banana Muffins	Zucchini Fritters with Jalapeño Popper Egg Cups	Chocolate-Covered Cherry Smoothie	Banana Quinoa Porridge
Lunch	Parmesan-Coated Chicken	Taco-Stuffed Avocados	Cheese-burger Salad	Garlic Lime Chicken	Juicy Turkey Burgers	Lentil and Quinoa Curry	Creamy Sweet Potato Soup
Snack	Chocolate Brownie Bites	Peanut Butter Cookie Dough Fat Bombs	White Chocolate Blueberry Fat Bombs	Key Lime Pie Fat Bombs	Chocolate and Sea Salt Fat Bombs	Butternut Carrot Ginger Soup	Everything Bagel Bombs
Dinner	Spaghetti Squash Pizza Bake	Spinach and Feta–Stuffed Chicken Breasts	Garlic Butter Salmon and Asparagus	Taco Pie	Decadent Crab Cakes with Lemon Butter Zucchini	Spicy Basil Chicken and Rice	Salmon Florentine
Dessert	Blueberry Vanilla Cupcakes	Lemon Cheesecake Mousse	Fatty Fudge Pops	Peanut Butter Chocolate Chip Blondies	Strawberry Cheesecake Pops	Wild Blueberry Vanilla Chia Pudding	Almond Clusters

One High-Carb Day

	M	T	W	T	F	S	S
	Standard Keto Diet	Standard Keto Diet	Standard Keto Diet	Standard Keto Diet	Standard Keto Diet	Standard Keto Diet	**High-Carb Phase**
Breakfast	Avocado Everything "Bagels"	Chocolate Coffee Chia Pudding	Buffalo Chicken Egg Cups	Chocolate Chip Banana Muffins	Zucchini Fritters with Jalapeño Popper Egg Cups	Vanilla Cinnamon Overnight "Oats"	Sweet Potato Fritters with Egg, Spinach, and Feta–Stuffed Peppers
Lunch	Parmesan-Coated Chicken	Taco-Stuffed Avocados	Cheese-burger Salad	Garlic Lime Chicken	Juicy Turkey Burgers	Greek Zoodle Mason Jar Salad	Quinoa Pad Thai
Snack	Chocolate Brownie Bites	Peanut Butter Cookie Dough Fat Bombs	White Chocolate Blueberry Fat Bombs	Key Lime Pie Fat Bombs	Chocolate and Sea Salt Fat Bombs	Vanilla Matcha Fat Bombs	Hot Chocolate Fat Bomb
Dinner	Spaghetti Squash Pizza Bake	Spinach and Feta–Stuffed Chicken Breasts	Garlic Butter Salmon and Asparagus	Taco Pie	Decadent Crab Cakes with Lemon Butter Zucchini	Baked Chicken Cordon Bleu with Twice-Baked Cauliflower	Bacon-Glazed Pork Chops with Applesauce
Dessert	Blueberry Vanilla Cupcakes	Lemon Cheesecake Mousse	Fatty Fudge Pops	Peanut Butter Chocolate Chip Blondies	Strawberry Cheesecake Pops	Wild Blueberry Vanilla Chia Pudding	Almond Clusters

STANDARD US/METRIC
MEASUREMENT CONVERSIONS

VOLUME CONVERSIONS

US Volume Measure	Metric Equivalent
⅛ teaspoon	0.5 milliliter
¼ teaspoon	1 milliliter
½ teaspoon	2 milliliters
1 teaspoon	5 milliliters
½ tablespoon	7 milliliters
1 tablespoon (3 teaspoons)	15 milliliters
2 tablespoons (1 fluid ounce)	30 milliliters
¼ cup (4 tablespoons)	60 milliliters
⅓ cup	90 milliliters
½ cup (4 fluid ounces)	125 milliliters
⅔ cup	160 milliliters
¾ cup (6 fluid ounces)	180 milliliters
1 cup (16 tablespoons)	250 milliliters
1 pint (2 cups)	500 milliliters
1 quart (4 cups)	1 liter (about)

WEIGHT CONVERSIONS

US Weight Measure	Metric Equivalent
½ ounce	15 grams
1 ounce	30 grams
2 ounces	60 grams
3 ounces	85 grams
¼ pound (4 ounces)	115 grams
½ pound (8 ounces)	225 grams
¾ pound (12 ounces)	340 grams
1 pound (16 ounces)	454 grams

OVEN TEMPERATURE CONVERSIONS

Degrees Fahrenheit	Degrees Celsius
200 degrees F	95 degrees C
250 degrees F	120 degrees C
275 degrees F	135 degrees C
300 degrees F	150 degrees C
325 degrees F	160 degrees C
350 degrees F	180 degrees C
375 degrees F	190 degrees C
400 degrees F	205 degrees C
425 degrees F	220 degrees C
450 degrees F	230 degrees C

BAKING PAN SIZES

American	Metric
8 × 1½ inch round baking pan	20 × 4 cm cake tin
9 × 1½ inch round baking pan	23 × 3.5 cm cake tin
11 × 7 × 1½ inch baking pan	28 × 18 × 4 cm baking tin
13 × 9 × 2 inch baking pan	30 × 20 × 5 cm baking tin
2 quart rectangular baking dish	30 × 20 × 3 cm baking tin
15 × 10 × 2 inch baking pan	30 × 25 × 2 cm baking tin (Swiss roll tin)
9 inch pie plate	22 × 4 or 23 × 4 cm pie plate
7 or 8 inch springform pan	18 or 20 cm springform or loose bottom cake tin
9 × 5 × 3 inch loaf pan	23 × 13 × 7 cm or 2 lb narrow loaf or pate tin
1½ quart casserole	1.5 liter casserole
2 quart casserole	2 liter casserole

Index